THE ESSENCE OF
TAI CHI

PAUL KERRY

Acknowledgments:

Photographic models: special thanks to Michelle Wattam and Doug Gerrard,
Tai Chi Practitioners.

Picture credits: p. 8, 9, 12, 14, 16, 23, 31 and 91 Charles Walker Picture Library.

Published in 2003 by Caxton Editions
20 Bloomsbury Street
London WC1B 3JH
a member of the Caxton Publishing Group

Designed and produced for Caxton Editions
by Open Door Limited
Rutland, United Kingdom
Editing: Mary Morton

Title: The Essence of Tai Chi
ISBN: 1 84067 305 2

THE ESSENCE OF
TAI CHI

PAUL KERRY

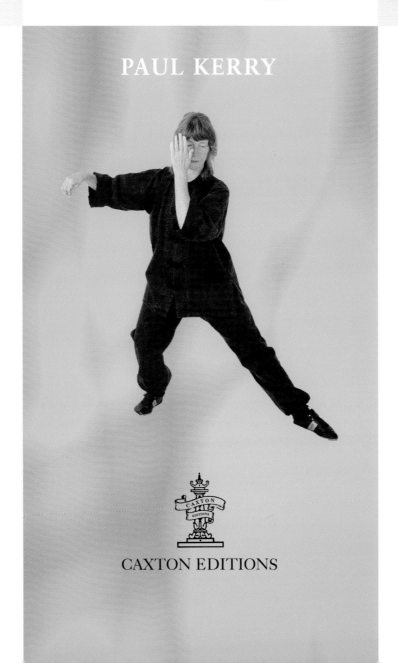

CAXTON EDITIONS

CONTENTS

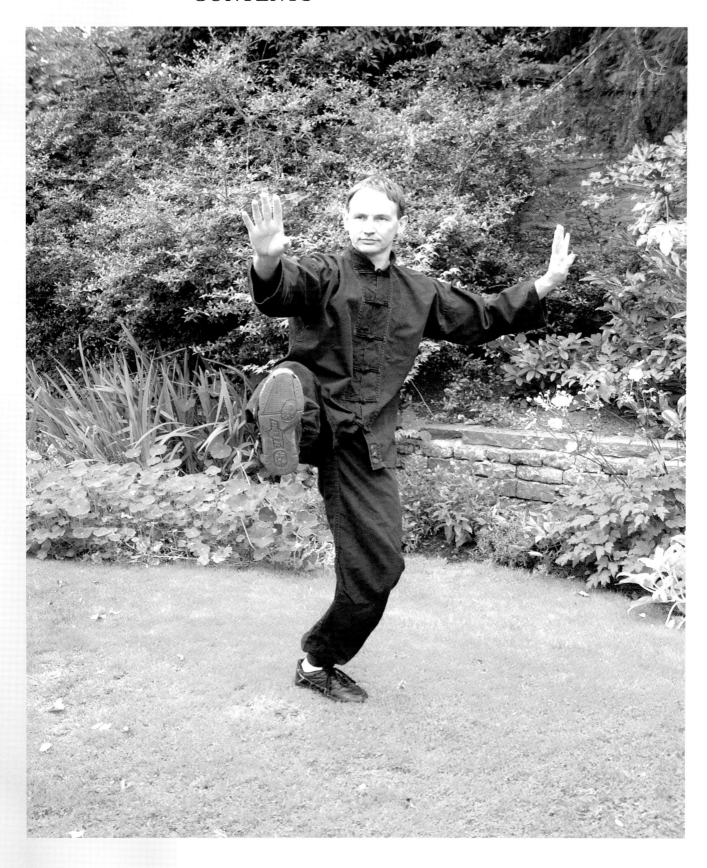

CONTENTS

INTRODUCTION

I n today's world more people than ever want to achieve greater fitness and better health. But they want to do it in a way that suits their present lifestyle.

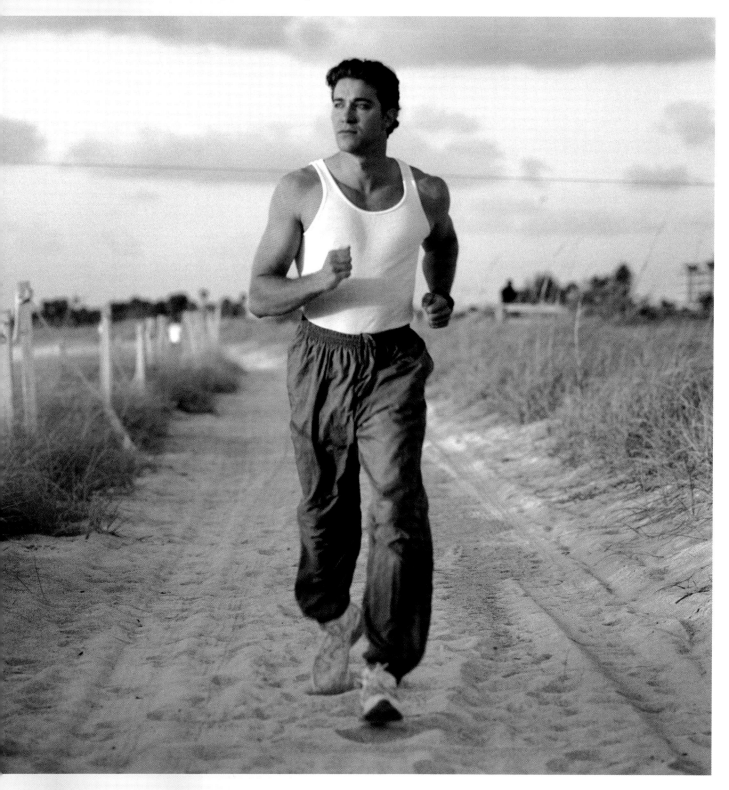

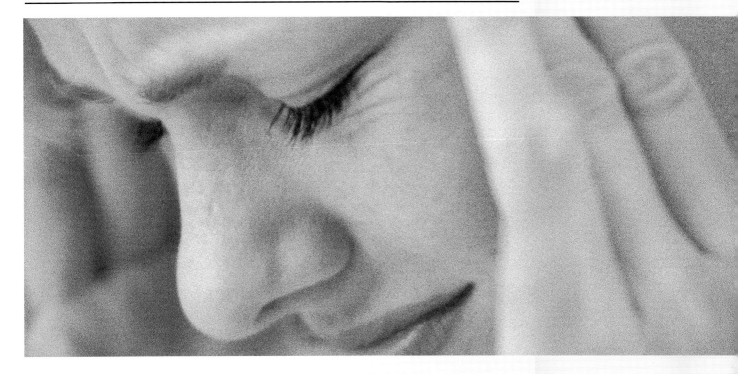

Who are these people? They are the old and the young, the fit and the less able-bodied, the poor and the wealthy, you and me.

What exactly do they want? Mainly relief and release from stress – seen as today's greatest impediment to leading a satisfactory life. Stress has a detrimental affect on our bodies as well as on our minds. It ages us and wears us down.

What are they looking for? Some countermeasure that they will be able to cope with, however old, tired, sick or weak they may be.

- They want something that they can do without having to exert even more of their depleted stocks of energy.

- They want something they can do on their own, at home. They want something that is not going to leave them hot and even more exhausted.

- They want something that they can do at any time that suits them.

- They want something that can be done in four or five minutes, but that can be extended, if they wish, to an hour or so.

- They want something that they can do regularly or periodically – every day or once a week.

Above: stress has a detrimental affect on our bodies as well as on our minds. It ages us and wears us down.

Far left: many people today want to achieve a healthier lifestyle but are scared off by the conventions which surround a so-called fitness regime.

Where will they find the answer to these questions? With Tai Chi, the exercise system that combines slow, graceful movements with calm, regular breathing.

What will they have to do? First learn a sequence of simple body movements. Then, practise them.

Tai Chi is defined by a series of postures, but the postures themselves do not constitute Tai Chi. It is the graceful movement from one position to the next, and the next, and the next that, when put together, make up Tai Chi. When performed correctly, the separate body positions combine to form one carefully choreographed, long movement that can best be described as balletic.

Tai Chi will benefit everyone. It is a gentle activity and safe for all. This is the reason why it has always been popular in China, where it originated, and why it is now sweeping the West. Tai Chi is a proven antidote to stress as well as a means of maintaining good health and feelings of relaxation and calm. It is not a cure-all. The wheelchair-bound won't be able to get up and walk after doing Tai Chi, but they will be able to cope with quite a lot of the exercises and will feel better for doing them.

Tai Chi is so gentle, relaxing and effective that it is also called by several more descriptive names: 'physical meditation' is one that suits it well, as does 'moving harmony'. Some of the names of the movements found in Tai Chi, such as 'face the tiger and return to mountain', 'white crane spreads its wings', and 'fair lady works with shuttles', illustrate the grace, fluidity of motion and serenity that exemplify the true spirit and nature of Tai Chi.

Below: Tai Chi when performed correctly can best be described as balletic.

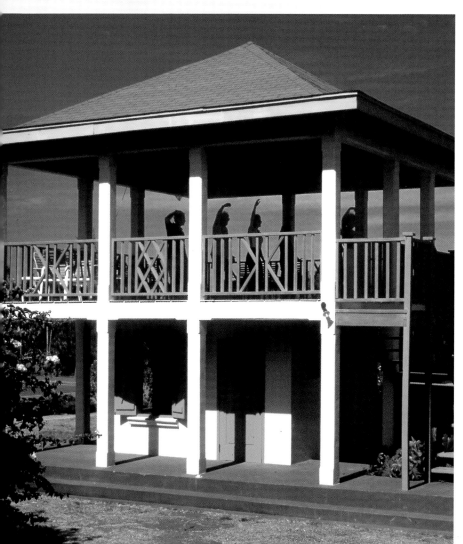

ORIGINS

The modern style of Tai Chi has evolved over many centuries, with some quite dramatic changes taking place along the way.

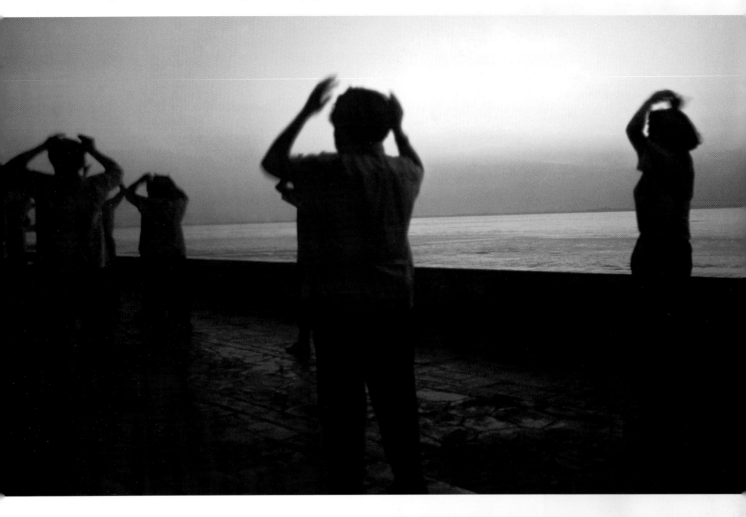

The full and correct name for Tai Chi is Tai Chi Chuan, 'Tai' being pronounced exactly as in the English 'tie', 'Chi' as in 'cheese' and 'Chuan' as in 'chew-on'. It began, as did so many Chinese exercise modes, as a martial art. The literal translation of Tai Chi Chuan is 'supreme ultimate boxing', or 'supreme unity of the fist', names which do little to describe the Tai Chi of today.

The first reference to what may have been Tai Chi is in a story told about Huang Ti, the Yellow Emperor, who lived about 2700 BC. It is recorded that he did special exercises for maintaining his good health, and that he based these exercises on his own study of the behaviour of animals.

Above: the literal translation of Tai Chi Chuan is 'supreme ultimate boxing', or 'supreme unity of the fist', names which do little to describe the Tai Chi of today.

A later account concerns a Taoist sage, Chan San-Feng, who lived in the 13th century. He had been trained in boxing and retired to a retreat for meditation. While there, he observed a crane and a snake fighting one another. What struck him was the grace with which the two creatures moved. The snake quickly but gracefully recoiled and weaved away whenever the crane attempted to attack with its bill, while the crane covered itself with its wings and fluently sidestepped whenever the snake attempted to strike with his fangs. It was the gracefulness of this fighting that impressed Chan San-Feng. There and then he decided to incorporate this elegance into a new style of boxing. Tai Chi Chuan was born.

As the centuries passed there was less conflict and less need for self-defence. But the exercises were not forgotten and evolved into the modern Tai Chi, as practised by millions of Chinese today.

Right: Chan San-Feng observed a crane and a snake fighting one another.

With time, different styles of Tai Chi developed. Some of these were short-lived but a few have remained in the Tai Chi repertoire. Most of these were advanced by different Chinese families and the family names were perpetuated in the name of the style.

Thus there was:

CHEN STYLE
HAO STYLE
OLD WU STYLE
NEW WU STYLE
SUN STYLE and YANG STYLE

Each style contributed some new aspect to Tai Chi that sought to be an improvement over former styles.

Today, the most common method is Yang style. This dropped some of the original faster, aggressive movements to leave the more modern, less energetic form of exercise that is acceptable to all.

Below: today, the most common method is Yang style.

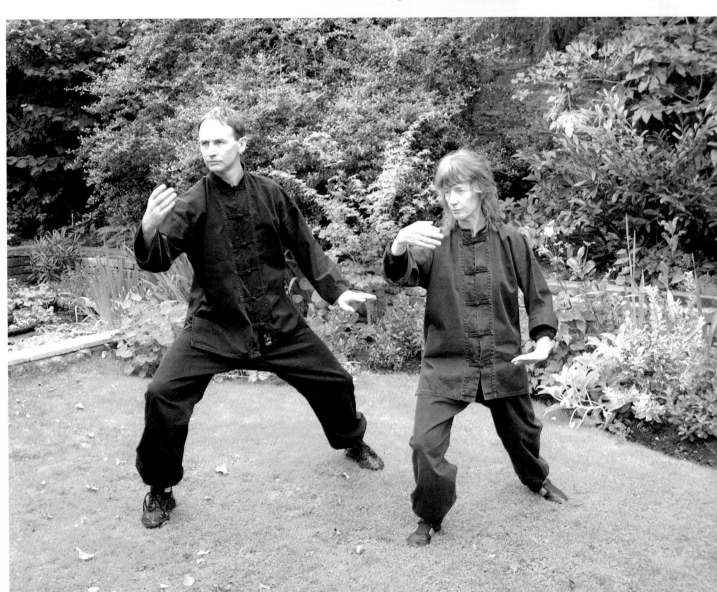

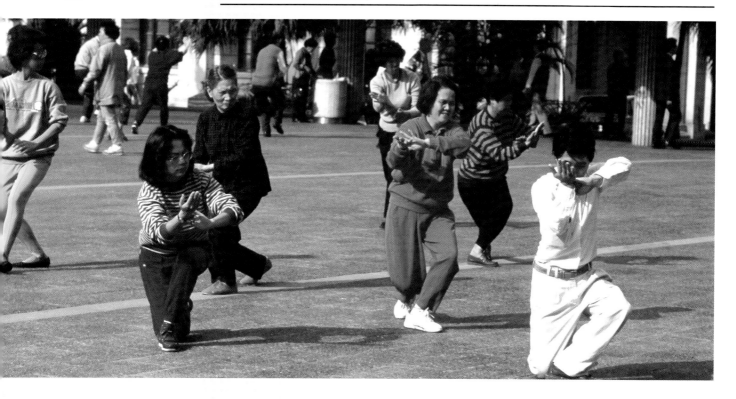

Above: what is suitable for a young, energetic man will be unlikely to answer the needs of an older, more sedentary woman.

Tai Chi is practised by performing certain groups of movements. As already mentioned, groups of movements have evocative names, such as 'Play the Lute' and 'Face the Tiger and Return to the Mountain'. Each position is then changed to the next by a fluid movement of the body, arms and, occasionally, feet. There is no pause between these positions, so that they join together into one long fluent movement. Each of these groups of movements is called a Form and there are many different variations. In fact, if you read up on Tai Chi, you will find as many different combinations of movements as there are books.

The simplest consists of about 20 movements, known as the Short Form. Different sets of movements lead up to the Long Form comprising as many as 108. To complete these Forms may take anything from a few minutes to an hour, depending on the number of movements, and can thus be tailored to individual requirements.

It is up to you to find the Form that suits you. What is suitable for a young, energetic man will be unlikely to answer the needs of an older, more sedentary woman. A person with more time to spare will be able to complete a longer Form than one who finds that time is at a premium. But one thing is certain – everyone will find a form of Tai Chi to meet his or her needs.

To understand how Tai Chi works, you first need to understand a little of the Chinese philosophy behind it.

The Chinese believe that, for good health, both the body and mind must be in harmony. There must be a balance between the two, with no stress on one side that would cause disharmony with the other. This is symbolised by the Yin Yang symbol.

In fact, Tai Chi is the correct name for this symbol, depicting a balance between the complementary but opposing forces to be found in nature. Thus, the symbols – light/Yang and dark/Yin – could represent day and night, cold and hot, male and female, and mental and physical. All are opposite to one another, but balanced in nature. The symbol is well chosen for, although it represents conflicting extremes, the curving boundary suggests change from one Form to the other, each tapering off as it appears to flow into the other. Also an integral part of Yin Yang is the eye of the opposite colour in the centre of the other half. This is called the seed and shows that even in the centre of darkness, there is the possibility of light growing, and vice-versa.

Balance is maintained by energy forces that are continually moving between the Yin and the Yang. This life-force flowing through our bodies in channels called meridians is known in Chinese as chi. If we are to maintain good health, chi will need to flow freely though all parts of our body. In Chinese medicine the mind, body, emotions and spirit are merely different aspects of a person and chi flows through them all. If any one aspect is upset, the balance of chi is disturbed and the person suffers. Any dis-ease – that is physical, or mental ill-health, however brought about – will cause imbalance and a block in the flow of chi.

Left: Tai Chi is the correct name for the Yin Yang symbol.

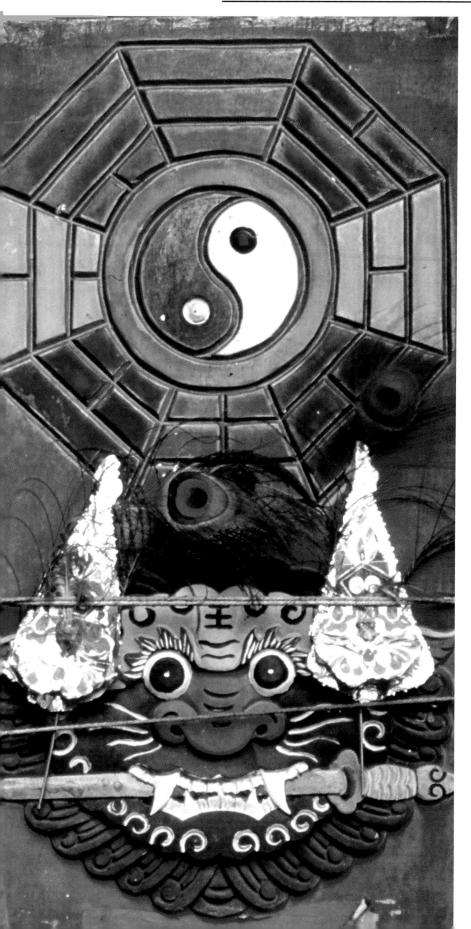

Tai Chi, with its subtle, graceful sequences, allows our bodies and minds to relax, and restores the balance by helping our chi to flow freely once again and re-establish health and vitality.

Put in physical terms, the simple movements of Tai Chi gently flex and then relax the muscles and tendons. This in turn fosters the flow of chi through the associated meridians. The chi then stimulates and invigorates the organs through which those meridians pass. At the same time, Tai Chi encourages the flow of blood through and round the body, so that it too can nourish all the tissues and organs. Because of the serene nature of Tai Chi the muscles are never tensed – any tension being unacceptable to Tai Chi – and thus the flow of both blood and chi is never restricted.

This then is the essence of Tai Chi. By encouraging chi to flow through the body a balance is created. Additionally equilibrium is established between mind, body and spirit so that they may work together as an integrated whole – as nature intended.

Anyone practising Tai Chi can look forward to the following improvements in their well-being:

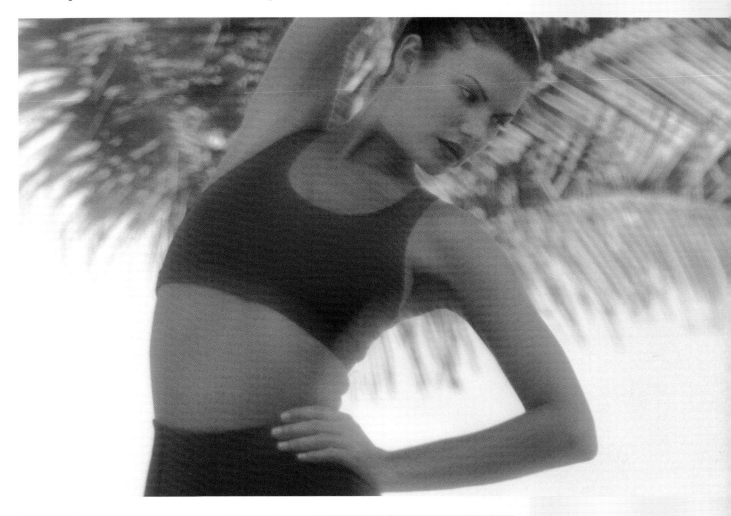

• An improvement in heart and vascular function – achieved as a result of aerobic movements promoting an increase in the body's oxygen intake. Blood circulation is increased with all the resultant benefits.

• Energy is increased due to the anaerobic effect mentioned above.

• Muscles in all parts of the body are strengthened. The arm and torso movements, together with the subtle weight transfer from one foot to the other, use muscles that may have lacked sufficient exercise.

• Relaxation and concentration are improved through the controlled breathing that is an integral part of Tai Chi.

Above: arm and torso movements use muscles that may have lacked sufficient exercise.

Far left: Tai Chi encourages the flow of blood through and round the body.

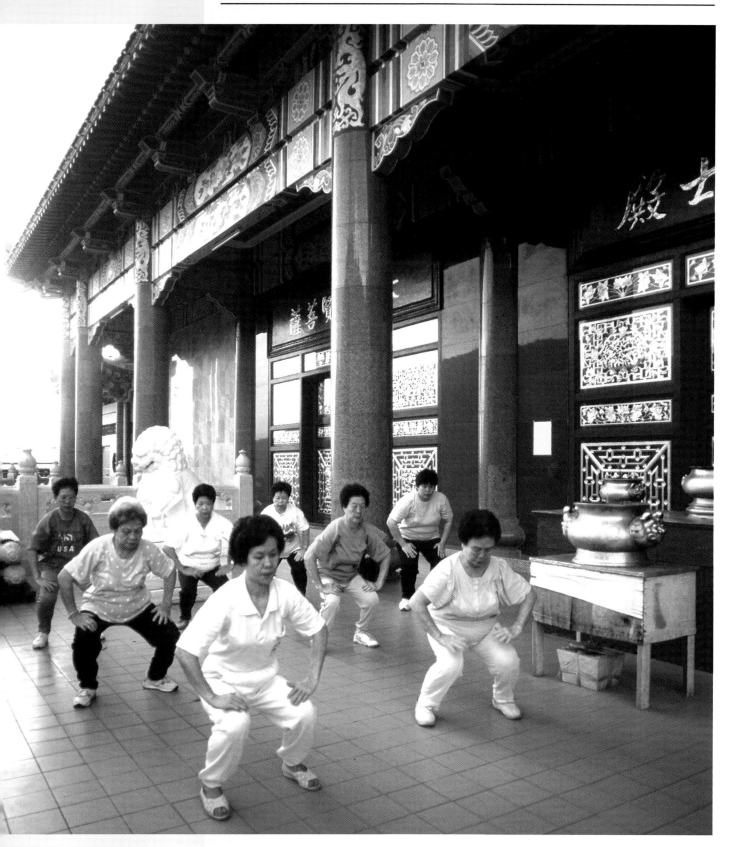

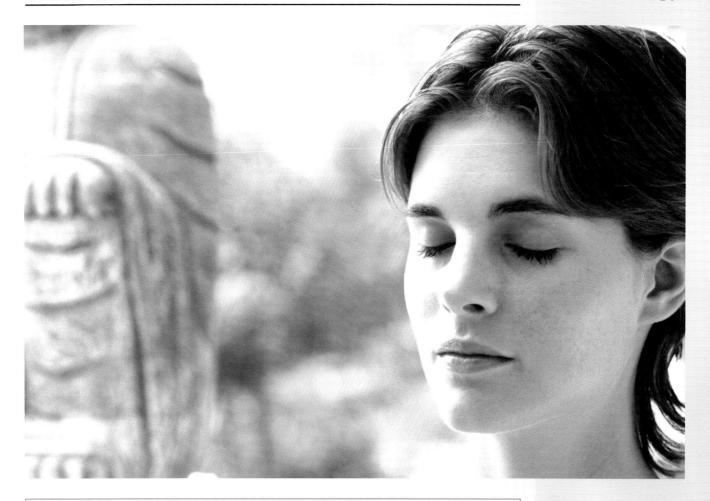

- Enhanced posture – as a result of being conscious of deportment.

- There is an increase in clarity of thought and the mind becomes more alert, yet relaxed. After learning the various movements, you will find that your mind can relax as you do them. Tai Chi has rightly been called 'meditation with movement'.

- An improvement in the sense of balance will be made. This is particularly noticeable in older people who are more prone to falling. The disciplined movement of the eyes, head and body at the same time resets the body's balance-centre to bring about this change.

- From a different perspective, you will feel more invigorated, more tranquil and more positive about your body and life in general.

Above: relaxation and concentration are improved through the controlled breathing that is an integral part of Tai Chi.

It would be worth while doing Tai Chi for any one of the above mentioned benefits alone, but it is the combination of all these points that is so effective in beating stress. The dynamic combination of all eight factors is a certain stress-buster. It is true to say that it is impossible to practise Tai Chi and remain stressed.

Related to stress, and another common ailment of today, is high blood pressure (hypertension). Records taken over the last 20 years show that this problem is on the increase, especially among younger people. About one in six adults suffers from persistent high blood pressure.

In most cases there is no known cause for this condition and the best cure is said to be a change in lifestyle. If this is your problem then there is no better antidote than a course of Tai Chi. Although this may not be seen as a change in lifestyle, it will completely transform the way that you look after your body and, if you look after your body, your body will look after you.

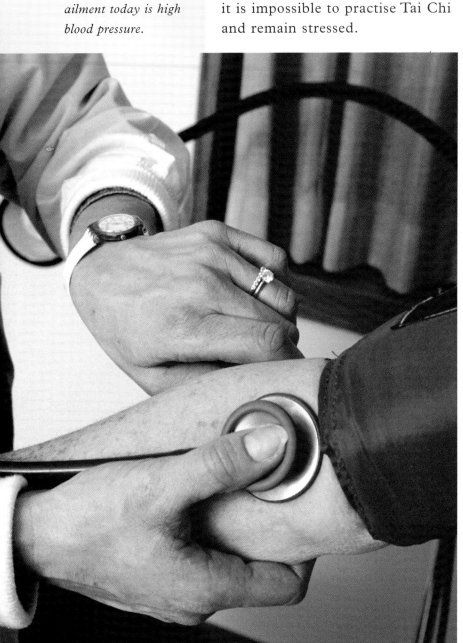

Below: another common ailment today is high blood pressure.

BEGIN AT THE BEGINNING – WU CHI

Tai Chi is usually undertaken early in the morning – preferably at sunrise – or at dusk. It is best performed outdoors and many maintain that it should be done near to trees – so that you can absorb the energy that they transmit. In China, where thousands practise Tai Chi at dawn, it is traditional to face south – the direction from which comes warmth and good fortune.

Below: Tai Chi is best performed outdoors and many maintain that it should be done near to trees.

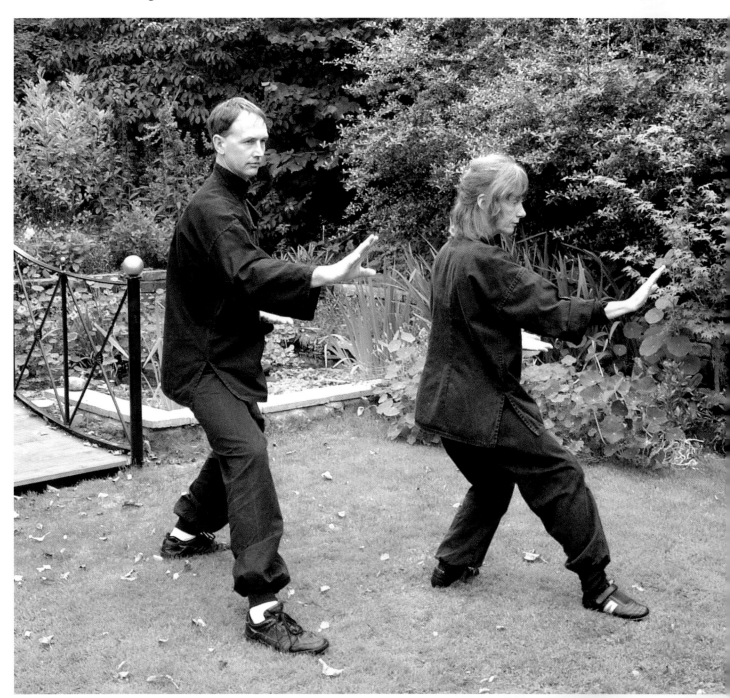

Below: relax, relax and again, consciously relax. This is the first basic principle of Tai Chi.

Your clothing should be loose and footwear soft, with no heels – the ubiquitous trainers are fine, though the traditional way is to be barefoot.

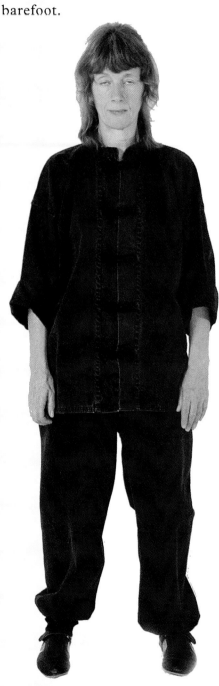

Learn the 12 principles and implement them whenever you are practising Tai Chi. They are as follows:

1 Relax, relax and again, consciously relax. This is the first basic principle. Chi can only flow through a relaxed body. Before you start your exercises, stand for a few moments and let any tension that you may have move down and out of your body through your feet. Feel your body become soft and yielding. This does not mean flabby and limp; it should be a dynamic relaxation. You are actively relaxing, not resting.

2 Having relaxed the tension from your body, it is time to relax your mind. Let go of all thoughts outside what you are now doing. Be in the present moment so that you are focused on the here and now. Concentrate on the idea that all your thoughts are going to be of Tai Chi and nothing else.

3 Stand with your feet shoulder-distance apart, legs and feet facing forwards. Make sure that your weight is equally distributed between your two feet.

4 Ground yourself. Imagine that you have taken root in the earth. At the same time you should claw the ground slightly, with your feet curling as though trying to grip the earth. Become one with the earth and feel that you are part of it, just as much as it is part of you.

5 Place the tip of your tongue at the front of the roof of your mouth, letting it rest lightly there as though speaking the letter 'L'. Close your lips and ensure that your teeth are not clenched together.

6 Stand upright, head held high, but allow it to tilt forward slightly, so that your chin is lowered. Keep your gaze on a level with the distant horizon and mentally smile. Remember that Tai Chi is meant to be relaxing and a pleasant experience. Some say that it should be done with a playful attitude.

7 Bend the knees slightly. This will remove any tension created by locking the joints. Though this posture may at first seem difficult and tiring, try to maintain it at all times. With practice it will become easier, and eventually quite natural to you. The bending should be only slight, so that the knees extend no further than above the toes.

8 When relaxing your shoulders, let them take on a slightly rounded position – forward and down.

9 Move the upper arms out, away from the body, so that there is space under the armpits. Imagine that someone has put a small ball under your upper arm and you are holding it there. The elbows are thus kept away from the body.

10 Bend the elbows slightly so that they are not locked.

11 Cup your hands as though holding a tennis ball, but imagine it to be made of meringue. Hold it gently, with no tension in the fingers or thumb so as not to crush it. Just let it rest there. The ball should be sufficiently large that it keeps the fingers slightly apart. At the same time, keep the palms facing in towards the body.

12 Finally, and of the utmost importance, you should be aware of your breathing. Breathing correctly is as important to the performance of Tai Chi as are the body movements and mental attitude.

Keep your mouth closed, if at all possible, so that you are breathing through your nose. Imagine that there is a lighted candle with the flame a couple of inches (50mm) in front of and below the tip of your nose. Breathe gently so that you will not extinguish the flame while exhaling or inhaling. If done correctly, this leads to a beautiful, steady flow of breath that is deeper and more controlled than usual. Practise this technique until you breathe so steadily that your imaginary candle does not even flicker.

Initially you may find that having absorbed these 12 principles, you are again tensed up. Don't worry; this is quite natural when learning something new. Just go through the steps again, repeating them until you are totally relaxed in mind and body.

The standing pose described is fundamental to Tai Chi. All the Forms start and finish in this position, which is called Wu Chi. Practise standing in this pose until it becomes so natural that you no longer have to think about it.

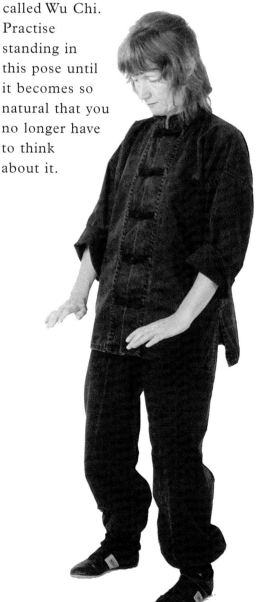

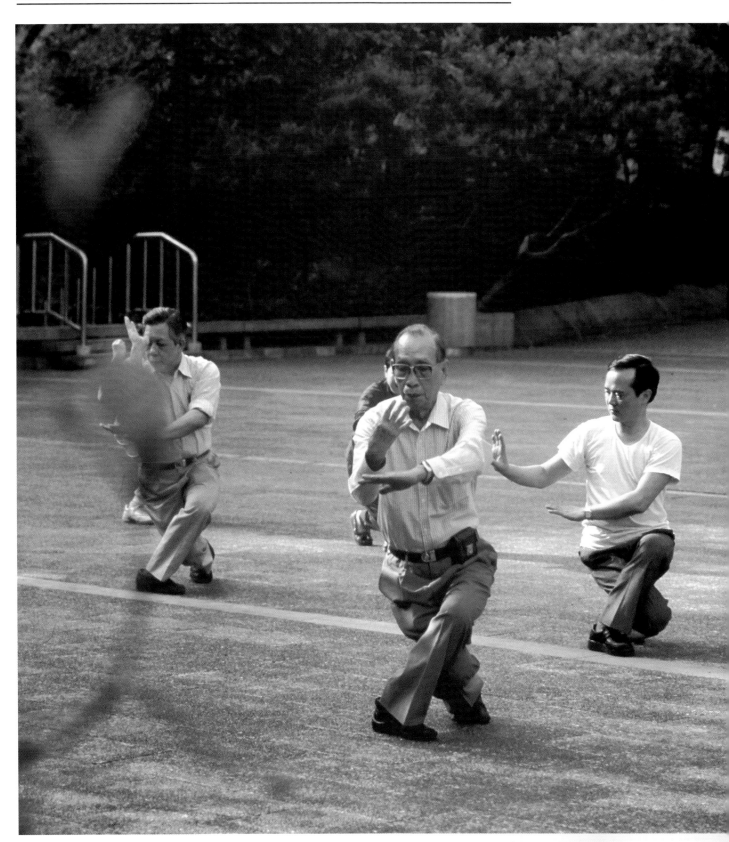

Unless you are used to undertaking a regular workout it is best to do some loosening-up exercises before actually starting to practise Tai Chi.

Right: Tai Chi, in the open air, Chen style.

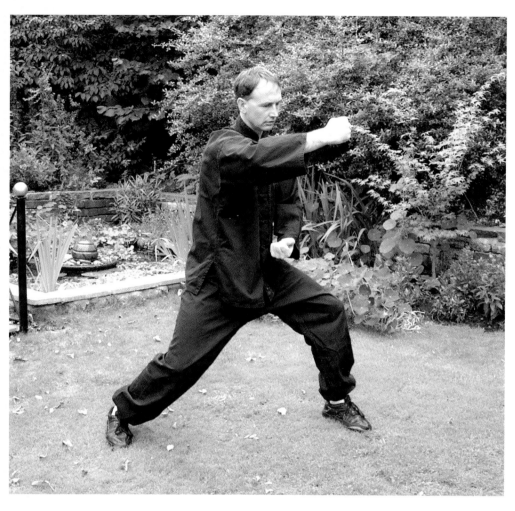

The following 12 exercises are quite simple and will take only a short time. They will ensure that you gain the maximum benefit from Tai Chi, and will not produce any side-effects. They are merely a means of loosening tight muscles. To attempt Tai Chi with tensed-up muscles would be counter-productive.

Dress as for Wu Chi and do these exercises in the open air if possible. Each of the exercises should be repeated three times, followed by a short rest before going on to the next. The temptation while doing some of these exercises is to close your eyes. Remember to keep them open, looking at one spot on the horizon the whole while. This will help you to maintain a good balance.

1 Stand in the Wu Chi position, consciously relaxing your mind and your body. Remember to breathe steadily and smoothly. Take three controlled breaths before starting the first exercise.

2 Lower your head so that your chin is resting on your chest. Then roll your head, unhurriedly but steadily, in a full circle, without forcing it. Breathe in as you start the rotation and out when your head is raised to its highest position, before it comes back round to its lowest position. Keep it rotating for three full circles, in time with your breathing and then stop. Pause for a moment then repeat this exercise, rotating your head three times in the opposite direction.

3 Stand quietly in the Wu Chi position and again become conscious of your breathing. As you start to breathe in, raise your shoulders into a tensed position, keeping your arms by your side. Hold your breath and your shoulders tensed momentarily and then, as you breathe out, lower your shoulders and relax them. Repeat, again keeping the movement in time with your breathing.

4 Now try to do the same exercise, but lifting your shoulders one at a time, and alternating them. The point of this exercise is to relax one shoulder while lifting the other.

5 Straighten your fingers so that they are pointing downwards, but without straining – like a guardsman standing to attention, though less stiffly. Now flex your wrists so that your hands and fingers point out, away from your body, while breathing in. Do this without moving your shoulders. Hold the position for a moment and then lower your hands back down while breathing out. After the third repetition, finish by shaking your fingers loosely as though you are trying to dry your wet hands.

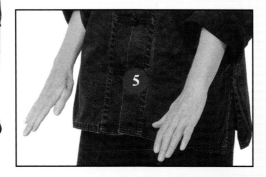

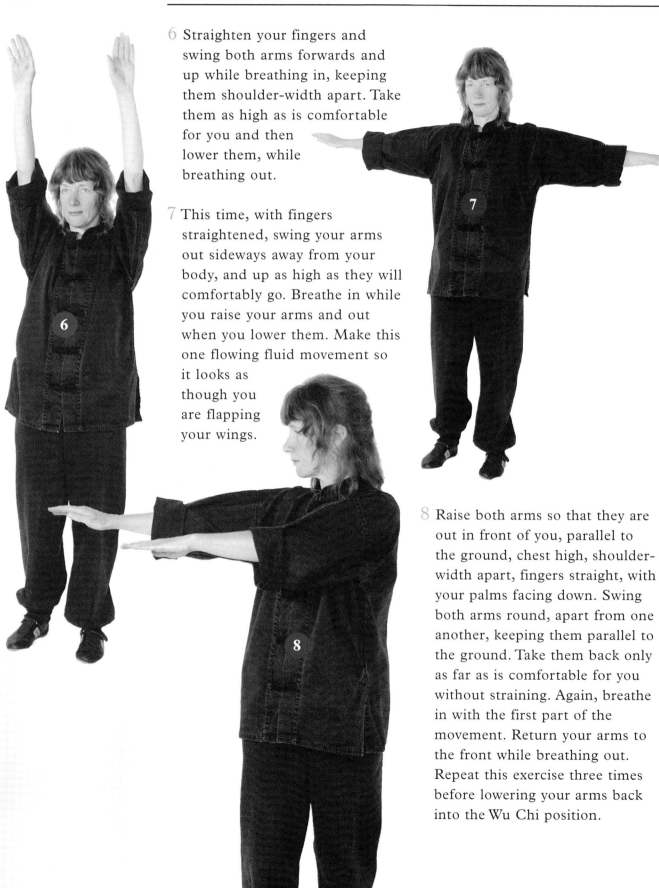

6 Straighten your fingers and swing both arms forwards and up while breathing in, keeping them shoulder-width apart. Take them as high as is comfortable for you and then lower them, while breathing out.

7 This time, with fingers straightened, swing your arms out sideways away from your body, and up as high as they will comfortably go. Breathe in while you raise your arms and out when you lower them. Make this one flowing fluid movement so it looks as though you are flapping your wings.

8 Raise both arms so that they are out in front of you, parallel to the ground, chest high, shoulder-width apart, fingers straight, with your palms facing down. Swing both arms round, apart from one another, keeping them parallel to the ground. Take them back only as far as is comfortable for you without straining. Again, breathe in with the first part of the movement. Return your arms to the front while breathing out. Repeat this exercise three times before lowering your arms back into the Wu Chi position.

9 Relax your waist muscles and those in your arms and shoulders, so that you droop forward. Let your arms swing in front of you. Don't strain – you are not trying to touch your toes. Simply relax, as though exhausted. This time you should breathe out at the beginning of the movement, hold the position momentarily and then breathe in as you straighten up. This is one exercise where you are not required to keep looking at the horizon. Let your neck muscles relax and droop with the rest of your upper torso.

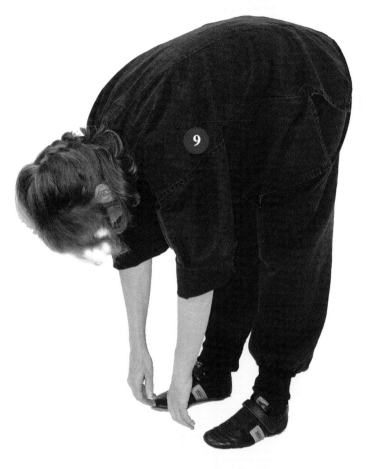

10 Keep facing forward and, without twisting sideways, bend to one side as far as is comfortable, letting your fingers trail down your leg. Breathe out when you do this. Slowly straighten up and breathe in at the same time. Then lean over to the other side and do the same, repeating the double movement three times. Try to keep this warm-up in one flowing movement, rocking gently from side to side.

11 Maintaining the Wu Chi position in all other respects, raise yourself on your toes while breathing in. Hold the position for a second and then breathe out as you slowly allow your heels to come back down to the ground. Avoid flopping back down – again the aim is to keep the whole movement elegant and flowing.

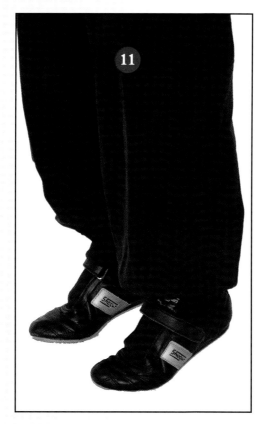

12 Finally, here is an exercise that is basic to Tai Chi and the Wu Chi position, and one that many beginners – especially those who are older – find most difficult. Raise your arms so that they are out in front of you facing forward with your hands shoulder-width apart. At the same time, keeping your spine upright, bend your knees as though you were going to sit down. Your arms will help you to maintain your balance, as will looking straight ahead. Take this exercise very gently and steadily and go no further down than is reasonably comfortable for you. Breathe out while sinking down, and in again as you slowly rise.

It is essential that while you are doing these 12 exercises you not only breathe correctly, but also that your mind is in tune with Tai Chi. Forget all your worries, cares and thoughts about the past and the future. Relax into the now. At first you will have to concentrate on what you are doing but, as this becomes second nature, don't let your attention wander. Notice the feelings in your body, how the energy is flowing through you and how you can put your whole self into each movement.

This group of exercises can be used at any time to help your muscle tone, poise, balance and attitude, but it is especially beneficial if done before each session of Tai Chi.

If you are a newcomer to Tai Chi, remember the following tips before attempting the Form.

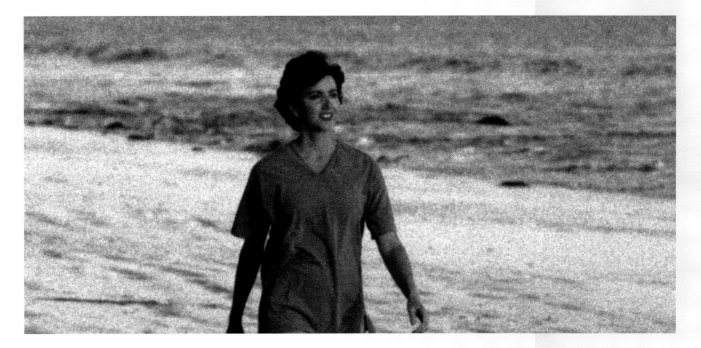

1 Relax, relax and, again, relax. This cannot be over-stressed or repeated too many times. Relaxation is not easy for beginners as they are still learning and trying to remember all that they have to do. With practice, the Tai Chi movements become more natural and you will not have to consciously concentrate on them. It is then that you will find it easier to relax. Until that happy moment, try to relax as soon as you become aware of tension, in body or mind.

2 Remember that Tai Chi is at all times a flowing movement, both physically and mentally. Learn to go with the flow, not forcing anything, even your thoughts. For the beginner, relaxing the mind and keeping it relaxed may prove one of the most difficult parts of Tai Chi.

3 The legs are the weakest part of the body as far as Tai Chi is concerned, and need to be concentrated on. Remember that the Wu Chi stance should be relaxed with the knees bent so that they are level with your toes. Initially it will be tiring to hold this position for a complete Form. Persist and gradually you will find that it becomes easier and less exhausting.

Above: learn to go with the flow, not forcing anything, even your thoughts.

4 Keep the spine and head upright at all times. This is not difficult to do, but can be hard to remember. Imagine that someone is very gently pulling your hair up from the crown of your head. You stretch your spine and neck to take the tension away, but without rising on to your toes.

5 We are all used to breathing in our own way. It is an automatic action, so it can be quite difficult to maintain the measured, smooth flow that is an essential part of Tai Chi. If you are at all tense, you will find that you tend to hold your breath. One way to ensure that you are not doing this is to listen to your breathing. You will soon find that the natural rhythm becomes so impressed upon your mind that you will immediately recognise any deviation. As you relax more and go with the flow, you will find that correct breathing becomes easier without the need to consciously think about it.

6 We are all used to observing all that goes on around us. When you start Tai Chi you will find it natural to watch what your hands are doing, to ensure that you are making the correct movements. Try to keep your eyes focused at some spot on the horizon. With experience you will find that this allows you to both relax and go with the flow, as it helps to avoid distractions.

Below: as you relax more and go with the flow, you will find that correct breathing becomes easier without the need to consciously think about it.

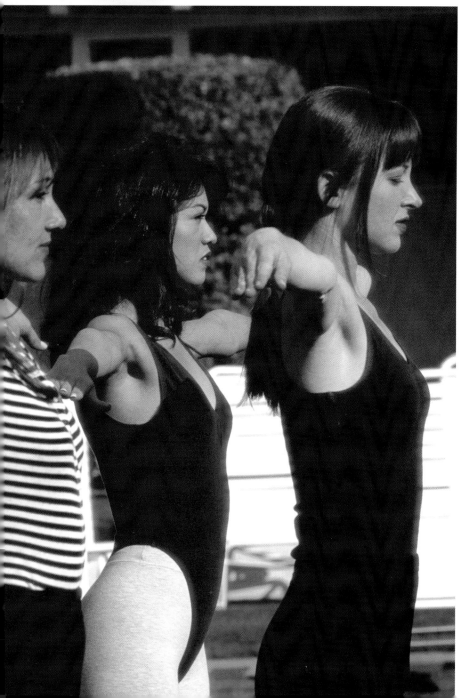

7 Never strain. If you have to do so then you are not performing the movement correctly. If your body will not allow you to make the full movement, go as far as you comfortably can. With practice you will find all the movements become easier – without straining.

8 On no account should you lock your knees or your elbows. The knees are the worst offenders here. Since we learned to stand upright we have, as a matter of course, locked our knees. This is why it is important to maintain the Wu Chi stance with the knees slightly bent. The aim is to keep the position as low as possible while keeping an upright back. When we extend our arms forward, as in many Tai Chi movements, we tend to lock our elbows. Remember to keep them slightly bent so that they cannot lock.

9 The Form, although composed of many different movements, should be performed as one uninterrupted, flowing action, like a well-choreographed ballet. It is also important to remember that you should keep moving at all times. There are no pauses or breaks in Tai Chi once the Form is embarked upon. As you learn it from the single still illustrations, imagine the fluid movement that will bring you to each position and how you will continue through to the next.

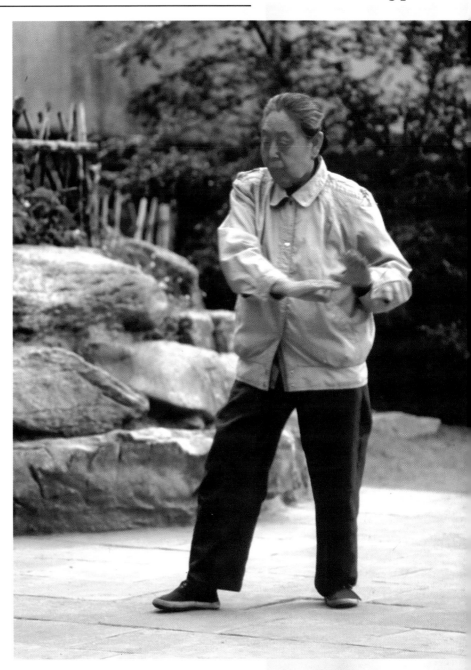

Above: remember to keep your elbows slightly bent so that they cannot lock.

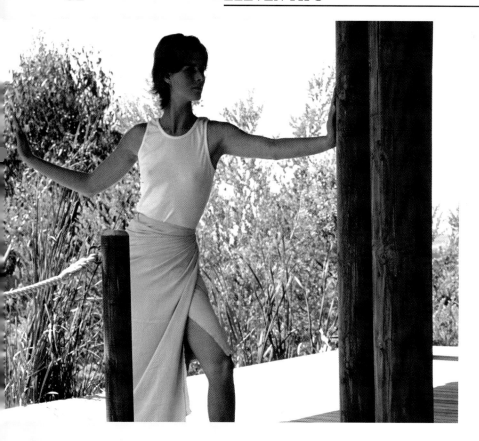

Above: imagine you are your arm and hand. Feel yourself, as a whole, moving extending, and reaching out.

10 In order to make your movements unhurried and smooth, imagine that you are performing them under water. Now you have that image in mind, go even further and change the water into a more viscous fluid – syrup or oil for example. Now imagine a dream sequence where everything, even your thought, is slowed down. As the TV presenters would put it – 'grab that sequence in slow mo'. All right, back to reality. Some Tai Chi classes are now being held in swimming pools. Try one if you can. You'll find it a vast improvement over water aerobics.

11. As you execute the Form, once you have learned the basic movements, you should try to alter your mindset. Try not to think of what the action is, and how to do it. Instead try to project your mind into the action. This is a difficult concept and is best explained with an example. If you are making a movement where you have to push your arm forward, think of it out there as an extension of your brain. It is not just your arm that is moving out; it is you, your mind, your understanding, your whole life-force that goes out. Imagine that, just for this one moment, you are your arm and hand. Feel yourself, as a whole, moving, extending and reaching out. This is not an easy principle to grasp and may be the last of your achievements in learning Tai Chi. But do persist with this idea. Once you manage it, you will realise what an important concept it is and how empty your Tai Chi was without it.

Obviously you will not be able to hold this book while trying to perform the movements of the Short Form. Try placing it on a stand or shelf. Prop it up at eye level, so that you can look at it while maintaining the correct head and eye positions.

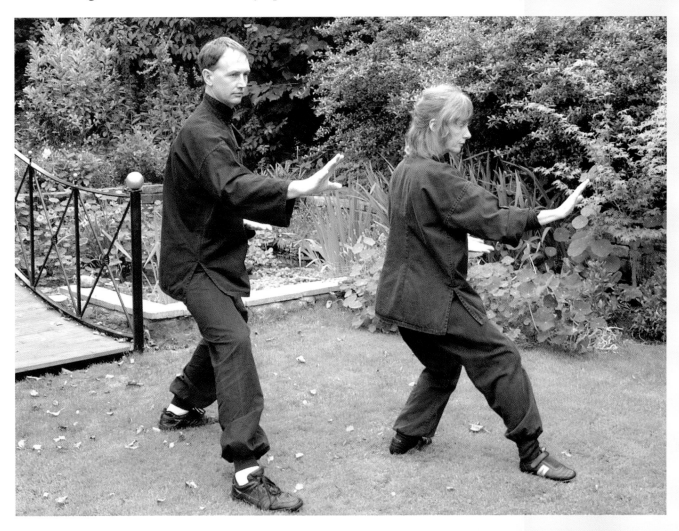

Another idea is to read the instructions given here, slowly, into a tape-recorder. Then simply follow the tape. When you perform the Short Form, try to do so in front of a full-length mirror.

By far the best method is to work with someone else. If you have a friend who is interested in Tai Chi, then you can work together. This is more fun as well as being an excellent way to learn. One of the main advantages is that, if you make a mistake, your friend can immediately stop you and help you to correct your error – something no cassette-player can do.

Above: by far the best method is to work with someone else.

Below: there is much more to learn if you are going to master the Long Form. This would be the time to attend a class in Tai Chi.

When, with the help of this book, you have mastered the Short Form, you will have some understanding of what Tai Chi is all about. But there is much more to learn if you are going to master the Long Form. This would be the time to attend a class in Tai Chi. A qualified tutor will be able to give you instant feedback as to how you are doing.

Watching others while learning is the traditional way in which most of us learn. This is how young Chinese children learn, watching their elders in the park each morning. With other students performing Tai Chi alongside you, the movements will be easier to follow, as you will pick up their steady rhythm. Also a professional tutor will be able to point up those nuances of position, breathing and thinking that need some small correction.

If you have difficulty in locating a class nearby, don't have a partner to work with or a tape-recorder, all is not lost. You can still improve your Tai Chi by using videos. These demonstrate technique and the Form. You may find them helpful and get the feeling that you are working in a group as you exercise in front of the television set. The disadvantage, of course, is that the video won't stop if you go wrong, nor is it able to correct you.

Finally, do remember to open the windows and get as much fresh air as possible.

The Short Form is a good starting point for beginners as it is quickly learned and takes only about 20 minutes to perform.

You may find that learning in the open air, where others can see you, tends to put you off. Start by working indoors, if you prefer, until you are sure of yourself.

The Short Form consists of 20 movements, but remember that, although they are described one by one, they are part of one smooth motion. An observer, knowing nothing of Tai Chi, should not be able to tell that you are performing an act that has been put together from separate units.

Some of the steps given may appear to be very short, while others are longer. The shorter movements are often no more than a means of linking one larger movement to the next. This is all part of the concept that the Form should be one continuous flowing action.

Each of the several movements has a different name. Some of these names are self-explanatory while others, to Western ears, sound rather exotic. They were given these names – for instance, 'holding a ball' – for two reasons. First, to help you imagine the correct movement and second, so as to make them more easy to remember. Although there are more modern Western names for some of these movements, I have, where possible, kept the original Chinese names to aid your imagination and memory.

This Short Form is almost standard and its full name is the Short Yang Form. Yang comes from the name of the family who devised this Short Form and has nothing to do with Yin and Yang.

Other teachers may have variations on this style, with different movements and different names for them. But basically you will find that they are all the same.

Left: each of the several movements has a different name – for instance, 'holding a ball'.

1.   OPENING

mind pictures

In front of you is a large bale of soft foam rubber. You are going to try to compress this bale by pressing down on it with both hands.

legs and feet

Both feet are kept, shoulder-width apart, in the Wu Chi position with the weight distributed evenly between them. As you press down, your knees should be bent as far as is comfortable for you.

body

The body is kept in an upright position, head erect, eyes facing forward.

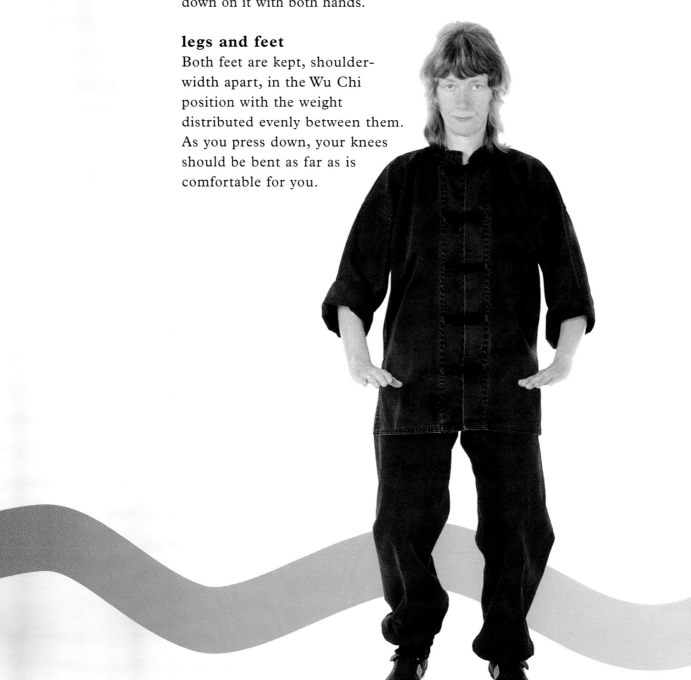

arms and hands

Raise both arms in front of you until they are outstretched, parallel to the ground. Keeping your shoulders back, turn your wrists so that your palms are facing down, fingers slightly apart.

Allow your elbows to fall back, keeping your forearms level with the ground and your hands shoulder-width apart.

Keeping your hands facing down, gradually straighten your arms, lowering your hands as you do so.

putting it all together

As you lower your hands, keep your arms straight. Bend the knees at the same time, until your hands are as near as possible to touching the floor. Hold the position for one second before reversing the body movements until you are once again standing in the Wu Chi position.

essentials

Avoid bending the knees so much that you are uncomfortable. You should not drop down to a position from which you cannot easily recover.

breathing

Begin the movement by breathing in as you raise your arms. Then breathe out as you lower them and allow your body to sink. Inhale again as you rise to stand in the full Wu Chi position.

let your chi flow

Envisage the chi in the palms of your hands as you press down. At the same time imagine the extension of your chi through your two feet, into the ground.

possible problems

Leaning forward as you push down. Remember to keep the body vertical. The best way to achieve this is to try to lean back, very slightly, as you reach down.

Remember that as you finish one movement it should flow straight into the next. You cannot go wrong if you simply move your body and arms in a natural way, maintaining the same steady rhythm as you use for the movements.

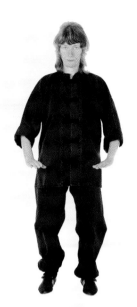

2.   HOLDING THE BALL

mind pictures
A large beach ball is suspended in space out in front of your chest. You are going to grasp this ball.

legs and feet
Adjust your weight so that three-quarters of it is taken on your left foot.

After moving your right arm, as described later, transfer your weight to your right foot and draw your left foot alongside so that your weight is once again evenly distributed.

body
Swing your body round a quarter of a turn to the right, pivoting on your right heel. Keep your head upright and looking ahead.

arms and hands
Bring your right arm up and out in front of you, bending the elbow as you do so, until it is level with your face. Your palm should be facing down.

Move your left arm forward and your left hand in towards your body at waist level. At the same time, turn your wrist so that the palm faces upwards.

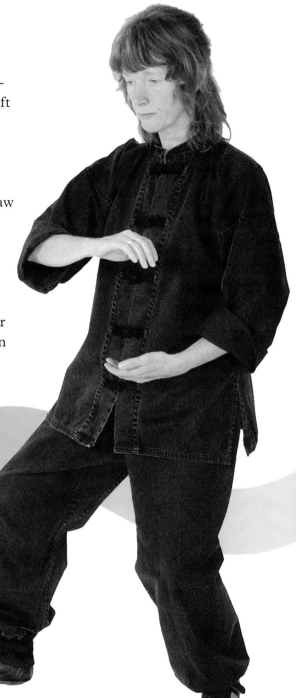

putting it all together

The movement of the left leg and right arm should be made at the same time, as should moving your right foot and left hand. As you complete the movement of your right hand, your left hand should already be starting to move.

essentials

Ensure that your palms are held one above the other and facing. If you imagine that you are holding a large beach ball, you will realise that your hands must remain a little distance from your body, to accommodate the bulk of the ball.

breathing

Allow your breath to flow naturally, in as you move your right hand, out as you move your left. The natural pace of your breathing will give you the timing for the movements.

let your chi flow

As you complete the move, you will feel the chi flow between your two hands, but don't hold them too far apart or the energy will be dissipated. Hold the position for a couple of seconds until you are sure that you feel that energy.

possible problems

Making the shoulders tense when completing the arm movements. Keep the shoulders relaxed and down.

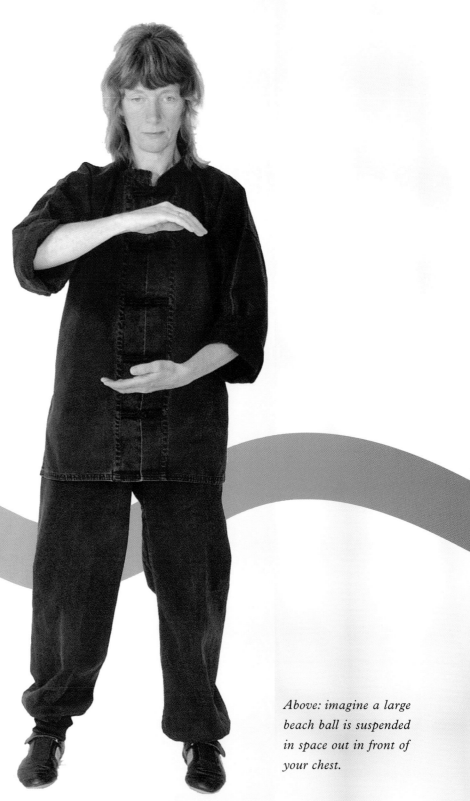

Above: imagine a large beach ball is suspended in space out in front of your chest.

3.   WARD OFF LEFT

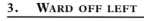

mind pictures
When performing this movement, imagine a swallow – a very light bird – landing on a branch that is gently swaying in the breeze.

legs and feet
Take your weight on your right foot. Slide your left foot out and away from you. Then bend your left knee so that your weight moves forward on to it.

As the arm movements are completed, move your weight back to your right foot and bring your left foot back alongside.

body
Turn your torso to the left so that you are facing in the same direction as your left foot.

arms and hands
Bring your left hand up level with the centre of your chest, palm facing inwards, fingers pointing to the right. Your hand should be about 12 inches (300mm) away from your body.

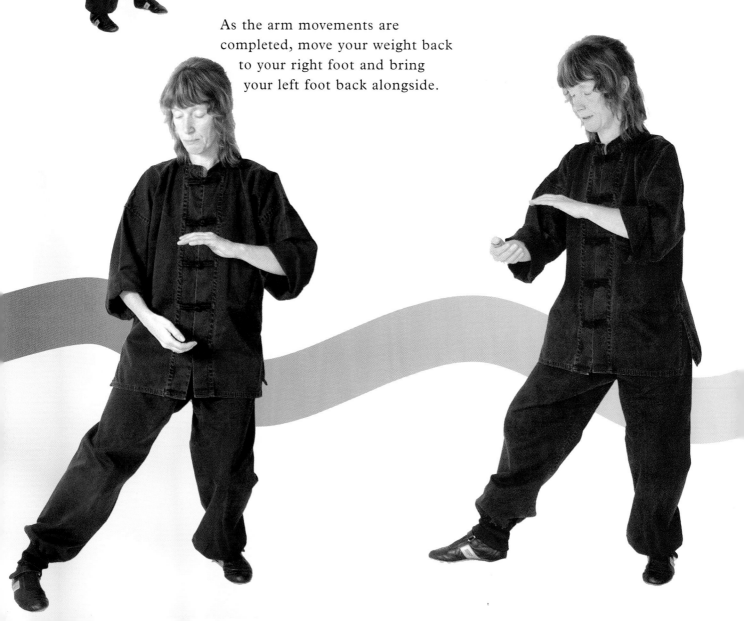

Lift your right arm forward, with raised wrist so that your palm faces out away from you and your fingers point up. Move it so that your hand comes between your left hand and your chest and you finish with crossed wrists, almost brushing palms as you do so.
In a steady movement, allow your right hand to fall back to your side, again almost brushing palms as it goes. As you do this, move your left hand until your fingers are in line with your mouth, pointing up, with your palm facing inwards.

putting it all together
This is all completed as one movement of legs, body, and arms. The name of this movement is obviously derived from a rather aggressive action that was used to repulse an attack on the person. The symbolism now used suggests the gentleness of a small bird, and your movements should be equally soft and graceful.

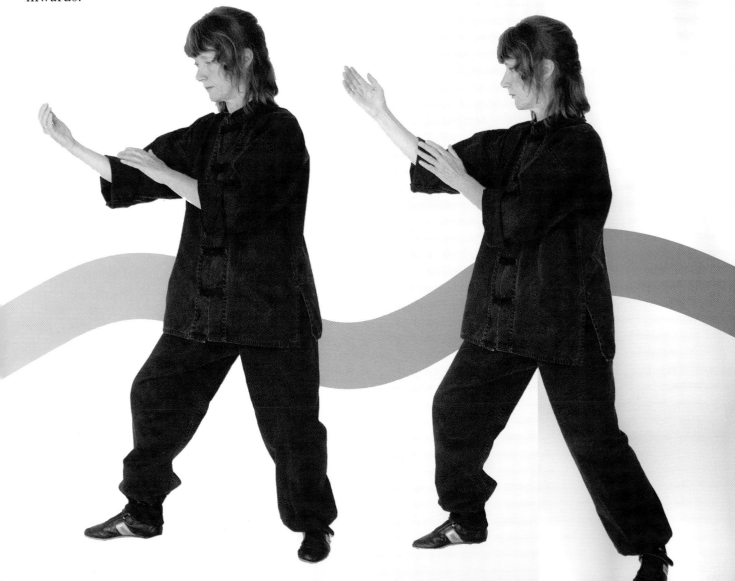

essentials
Keep the body upright, the arms relaxed. Even when the arms are curved up to the chest, the shoulders, elbows, wrists and fingers should have no tension in them.

let your chi flow
When both arms are raised, you will feel the chi flow quite strongly between your two hands. Maintain the flow for a few seconds before completing the move.

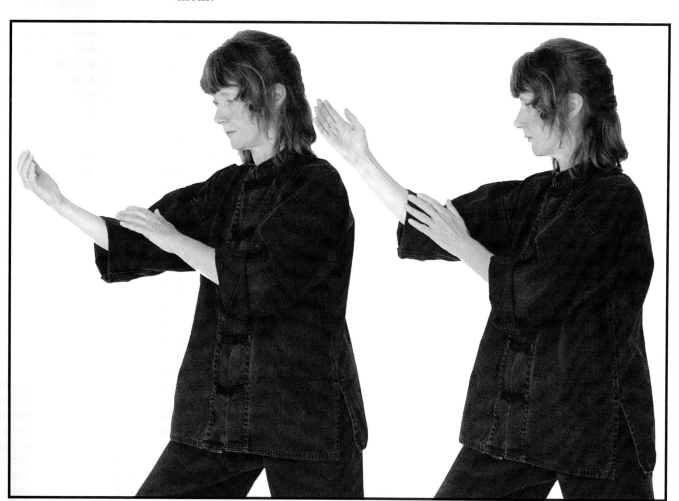

breathing
Pick up the point where you are naturally breathing in to start the movements. Complete the in-breath with the upward movements and then breathe out as your right arm falls away.

possible problems
Initially, you may be tempted to make the movements separately and thus lose the whole body-rhythm that is essential here.

4.   GRASPING THE BIRD'S TAIL

mind pictures

For this movement imagine that you have a bird perching on your left wrist. You stroke it with your right hand, starting at its head, and ending down at its tail. This is obviously a rather large bird and it's best to picture in your mind's eye something like the crane that will be mentioned later. As you finish stroking the bird, it takes wing and flies away.

Below: for this exercise it is best to picture in your mind's eye something like the crane.

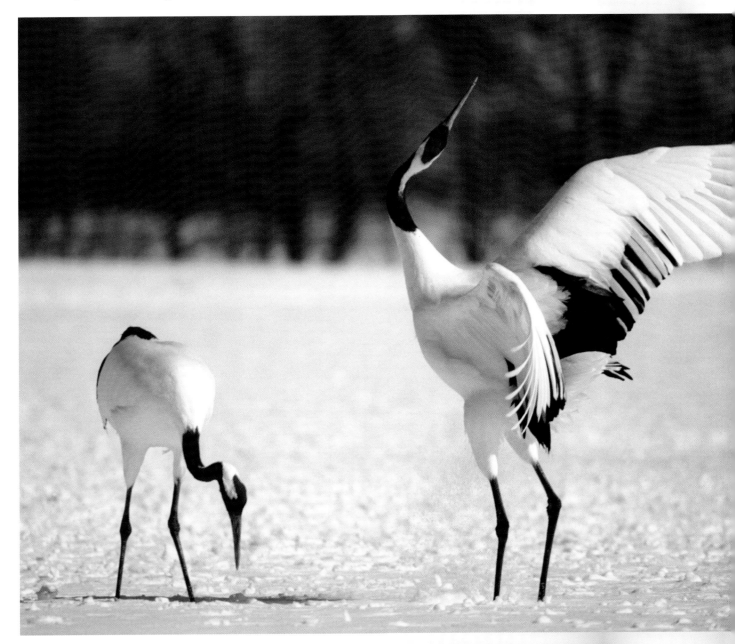

legs and feet

Take three-quarters of your weight on your left foot. Then pivot on your right foot, keeping your heel on the ground and the ball of your foot raised.

body

Turn your body to the right, one-quarter of a turn.

arms and hands

Bring your right arm up to your chest, just below your throat, with the palm facing down and your fingers pointing to the left.

Bend your left elbow until your lower arm is parallel to the ground, pointing forward away from you. Your left hand should be level with your waist, palm down.

Sweep your right hand down and away to the right, to hip level, palm down and fingers pointing forward.

As your right hand falls away, move your left hand up, keeping the palm facing in.

putting it all together

If you maintain the mind picture above, the correct flow of movements will automatically fall into place. It is important to actually feel the bird – feel the resistance under your right hand, and the weight of the bird on your left arm.

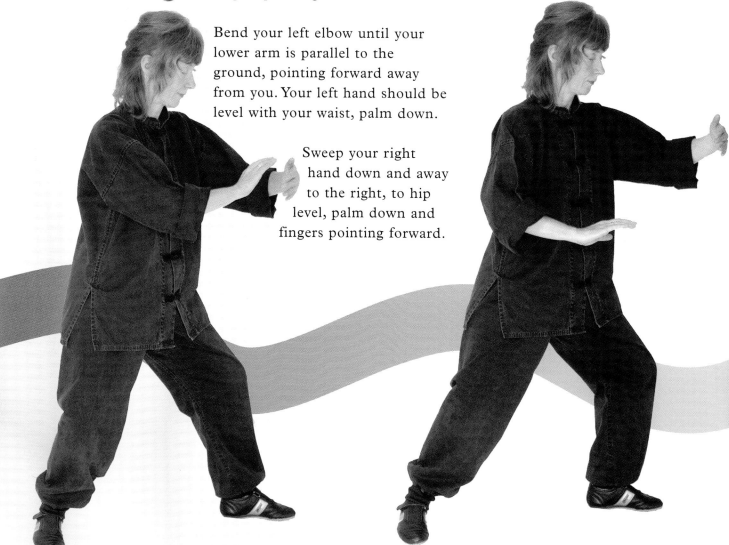

essentials

All the movements should be accomplished together – weight and foot movement, right arm and left arm rising. This must be one flowing movement where all the elements are integrated at the same time.

breathing

Breathe in as you raise your arms. Exhale a long sigh as your right arm falls away and the bird flies off. Again, the steady pace of your breathing should dictate the speed at which you carry out the movements.

let your chi flow

The chi should flow through the right palm as it sweeps down and away. It should also be felt, at the same time, in the left forearm.

possible problems

Beware of letting your eyes follow the movements of your right hand. Instead, watch the bird after it has left your wrist and follow its flight as it wings away to the horizon.

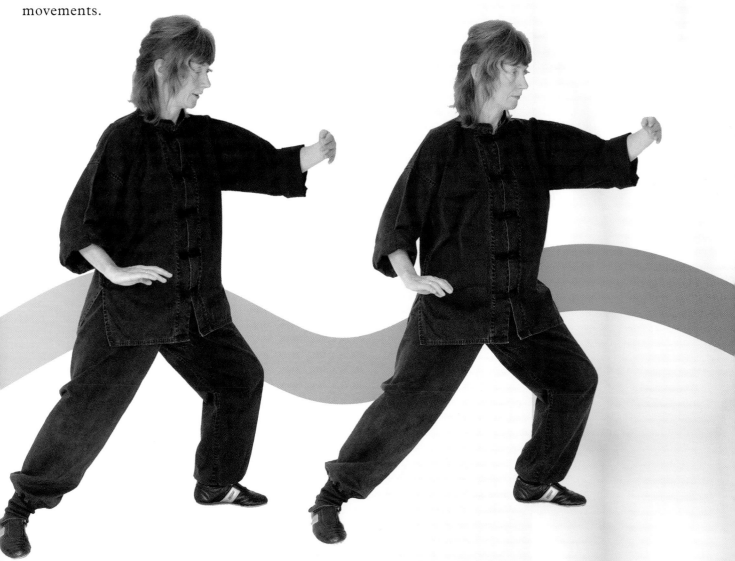

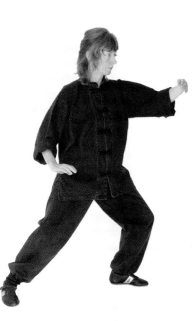

5. ROLL BACK

mind pictures
This title is used to describe the movement of your hands as they pass across your body. Picture the ocean waves rolling back from the shore.

legs and feet
Start with your weight on your right foot. As your arms come forward, move your weight back onto your left foot. Then, as you complete the movement, shift your weight back to your right foot.

body
Twist your body at the same time as you move your feet so that you swing to the right to start with and then back to the left as the move is completed.

arms and hands
Bring your left hand up across your body, with your palm open, facing up so that it almost cups the right elbow.

Reach up and out with your right hand, following the line of your right foot. As you do so, move your right hand, from the wrist, in a complete circle.

At the same time that you transfer your weight back on to your right foot, sweep both arms down back to your sides.

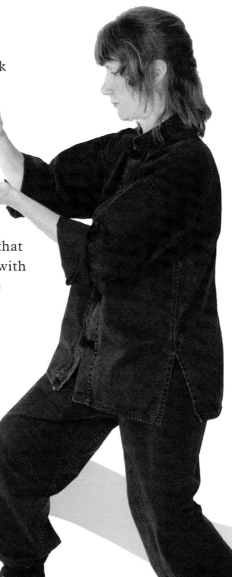

putting it all together

During this movement, move your arms, hands and legs all at the same time. No part of the body should be static during the roll back.

essentials

While concentrating on the arms, don't forget that, although your weight is transferred from one leg to the other and back again, your knees should not be locked at any point.

breathing

Time the movement so that you start while breathing in. As your right arm is extended, push the air out as you exhale so that the two pushing movements are combined.

let your chi flow

Feel your chi flow through your right hand as it circles and then through your feet into the earth as your hands come back to your sides.

possible problems

Avoid the tendency to lean forward as you push your hand forward. Ensure that you keep your palm flat and your fingers straight but slightly spread as you circle your right hand.

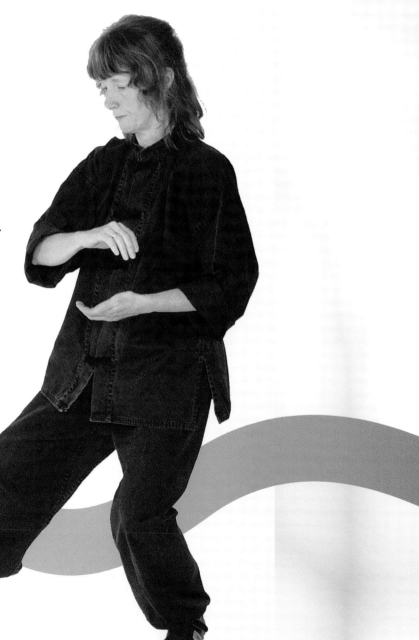

6. PRESS RIGHT

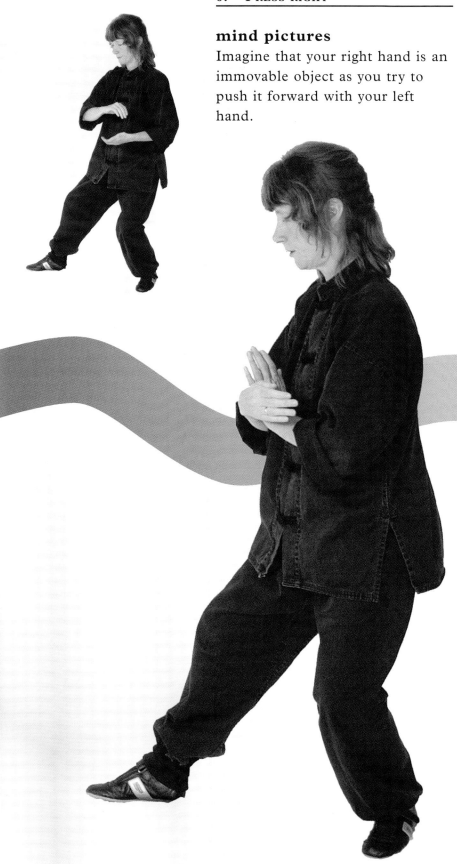

mind pictures
Imagine that your right hand is an immovable object as you try to push it forward with your left hand.

legs and feet
When the pressing begins, your weight should be transferred on to your left foot as you swivel to the right on your left heel.

body
The body remains static until you press forward and then it swings naturally to the right.

arms and hands
Bend both elbows and bring your arms across your body and up, so that they are crossed at the heel of your hands. Your palms should be facing, fingers straight and slightly apart, right hand on the inside, palm facing out and right hand on the outside, palm facing in. When they are together, start to press forward with your left wrist. Resist this pressure by holding your right arm in position, but allow the push to twist your body to the right.

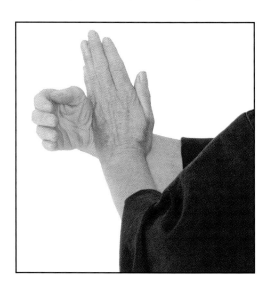

putting it all together

There is one nearly static moment here as you press the heels of your hands together, but it is only the hands that are stationary. As your hands come together and you twist your body, there should be no problem with making this press one flowing movement.

essentials

Keep your head upright and your eyes on the horizon.

breathing

Breathe in as you raise your arms, out as you press, and in again as you finish the movement.

let your chi flow

As you bring your hands together you will feel the chi flow between them. Then when you begin to press them together feel the energy coming up from the ground, through your right leg and through your body to your left hand.

possible problems

As you press your hands together you may tense your whole body. While there is bound to be pressure in your elbows and shoulders, try to keep the rest of your body relaxed.

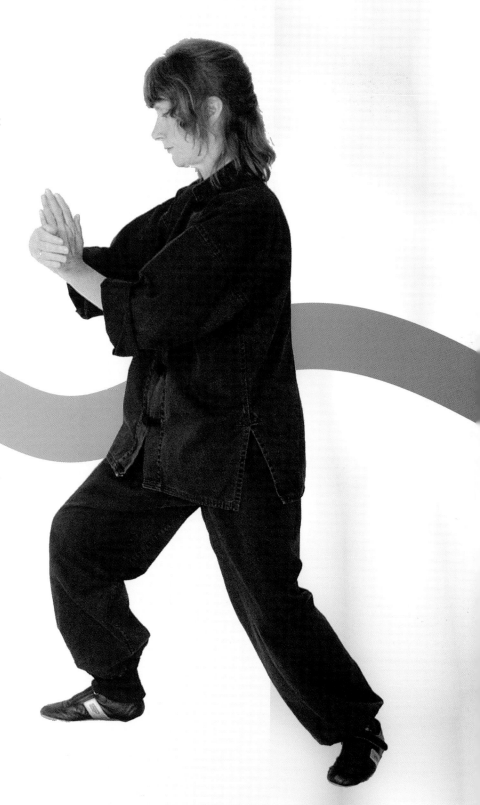

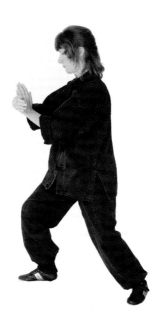

7.   OPEN

mind pictures

Imagine that you are opening your arms to embrace the whole universe. This is a very short movement that ensures a smooth transition from the previous movement to the next.

legs and feet

Maintain your feet and weight as they were at the end of movement 6. *Press Right*

body

Your body similarly maintains the same position as at the end of movement 6. *Press Right*

arms and hands

Move your arms so that they open out in front of you. Move your hands so that they are in line with your forearms, shoulder-width apart, fingers straight but not tense. Keep the elbows bent and slightly in front of your waist.

putting it all together
As only arm movements are involved, the action should flow freely and naturally.

essentials
This open move is designed to assist with a smooth transfer from the previous movement *(6. Press Right)* to the next *(8. Push Left)*.

breathing
Inhale after the last press and exhale as you open your arms.

let your chi flow
Feel the chi flow from both hands as you open your arms.

possible problems
As this is such a short movement there is a tendency to rush it. Take it steadily and smoothly just as with any other movement. Let your breathing dictate the pace.

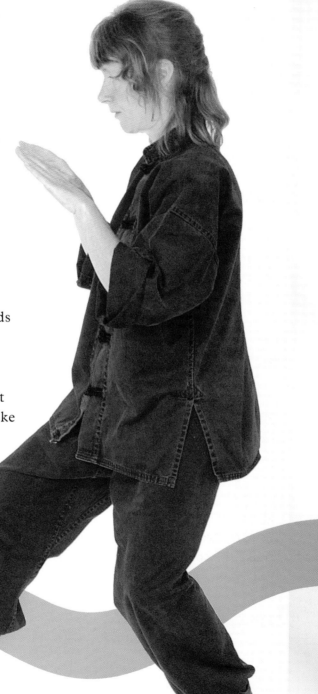

8.   PUSH LEFT

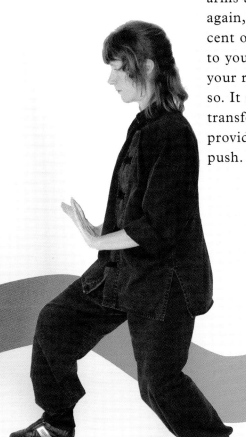

mind pictures
Imagine that you are standing in front of a large, heavy, wooden door that has rusty hinges. You must push it with both hands to close it.

legs and feet
Move 75 per cent of your weight to your left foot, bending the knee as you do so.

As the arms are moved up, shift your weight back on to your right foot.
When, later in the movement, your arms are moved forward again, transfer 90 per cent of your weight back to your left foot, raising your right heel as you do so. It should be this weight transfer that provides the push.

body
Turn your upper body so that you are facing out over your left foot. Keeping the body upright, allow it to move back and then forward as your weight is transferred from one foot to the other.

arms and hands
Drawing your elbows back, straighten them slightly so that your hands come down level with your hips. Keep your hands facing forward so that you will not bring them back too near your body.

Push both arms forward and up to chest height, as though closing the door. As you push, remember to keep your arms slightly bent so that the elbows are not locked.

putting it all together

Keep in mind the picture of closing the door. Note that this is not a straight push with the arms; the push should come from the legs and feet in the relocation of your weight.

essentials

Ensure that it is the movement of the body, through the legs, that pushes the hands forward. Make the body and arm movements at the same time. Remember to keep the body upright the whole time, head erect, looking straight ahead.

breathing

Take a steady breath in as you lower your arms and then exhale in time with your push forward.

let your chi flow

Feel the chi flow from both hands as you push forward.

possible problems

Leaning the body back and then forward is the temptation here – to be avoided at all costs if the movement is to be made correctly. Also remember not to allow your knees to lock at any point, even at the end of the movement when you are pushing forward.

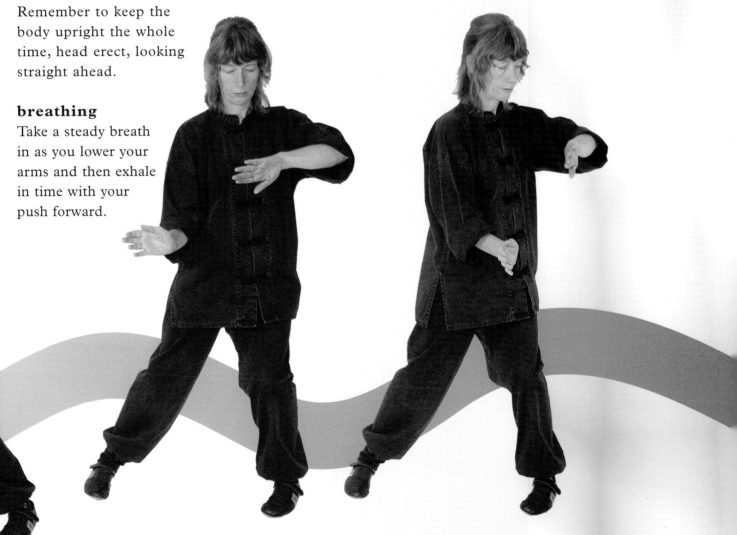

9.   SINGLE WHIP TO THE LEFT

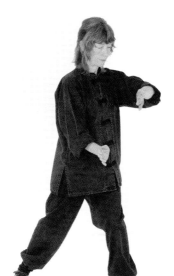

mind pictures

While performing *The Whip* imagine a willow tree blowing and bending in the breeze. Move with that same gentle motion that is never hurried or jerky. This movement may appear to be long and complicated. This is not so – it is simply that more detail has been given in order to help you. The name of the movement, *The Whip*, belongs to the time when Tai Chi was a true martial art.

legs and feet

Begin with your feet at shoulder distance apart. As you start the arm movements,transfer all of your weight on to your left foot and lift your right foot so that it is just clear of the ground. Swivel your right foot so that the toes are pointing in, towards your left foot. Place it down still putting little or no weight on it.

Gently bend both knees as though you are preparing to sit down.

Move 75 per cent of your weight back on to your right foot for the end of the movement.

body

Body movement from the waist follows the arm movements so that your shoulders swing round 45 degrees to the left.

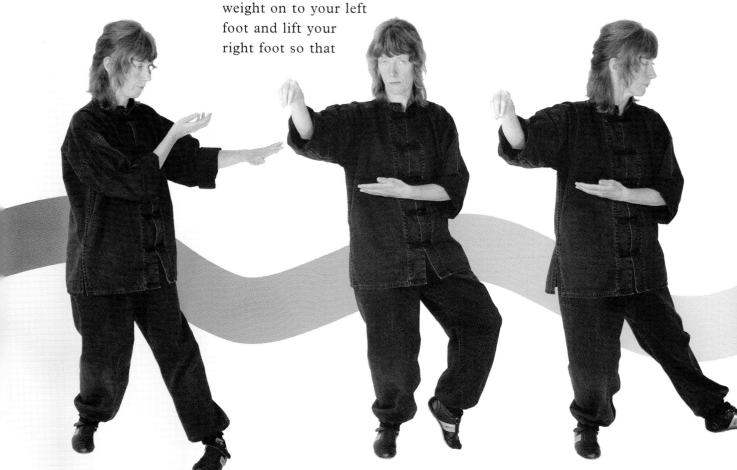

arms and hands

Draw back your hands from the push, so that your elbows are bent, maintaining their former height.

Push your left elbow out to the side and turn your left wrist so that your palm is facing left. At this point your hand should be level with your shoulder, while your elbow is dropped lower.

Your right arm should be still extended with palm facing forward.

Swing both arms round to the left as you swivel at the hips. As you do this, raise your right arm and at the same time make a hook with your right hand.

This is done by closing the palm so that your fingertips touch your thumb, while dropping the wrist.

As you return your weight to your right foot, almost straighten your right arm and raise it out and up, level with your head.

At the same time swing your left hand and arm out to the left.

Finish by allowing your right hand to come back until it is level with your heart, turning the wrist so that the palm is facing out away from your body with the thumb pointing down.

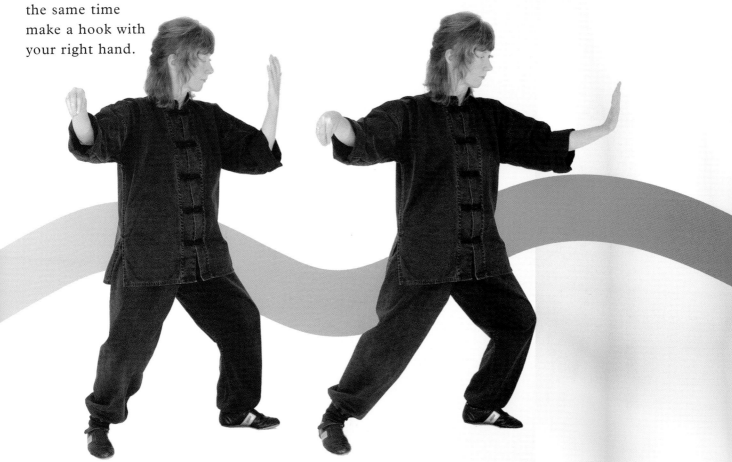

putting it all together

At first this may seem an awkward movement; with practice it can become one of the most elegant movements of the Short Form.

essentials

Remember that this is one complete flowing motion. Avoid a tendency to close in the arms. Keep them open – remember the small ball that you are holding under each armpit.

breathing

Although there are more movements in *The Whip* than in the previous sections, they are all accomplished within one inhalation and exhalation. Breathe in as you start the movement. The out-breath should come as you swing to the left. As always, the natural breathing gives you an idea of the timing for the whip.

let your chi flow

Again you will feel the chi flowing through both hands, particularly in the parts of the movement where your arms are extended, and also through whichever foot is supporting your weight at the time.

possible problems

The most common difficulty here is coordinating all the movements into an integrated whole. The variety of movements means that there is the likelihood of concentrating on one action and allowing other parts of the body to become tense.

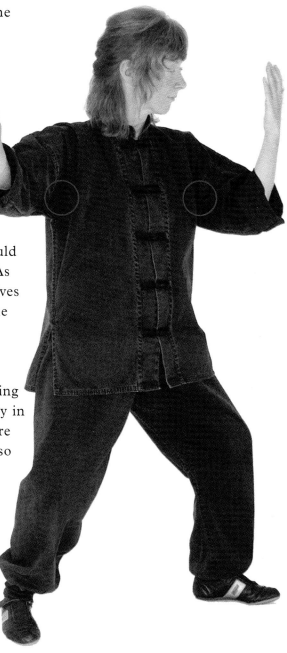

10. PLAY THE LUTE RIGHT

mind pictures

The lute is a guitar-like instrument with a long neck and a pear-shaped body, much used from the 14th to the 17th centuries.

In *Play the Lute*, imagine that your right hand is supporting the neck of the instrument while the left strums.

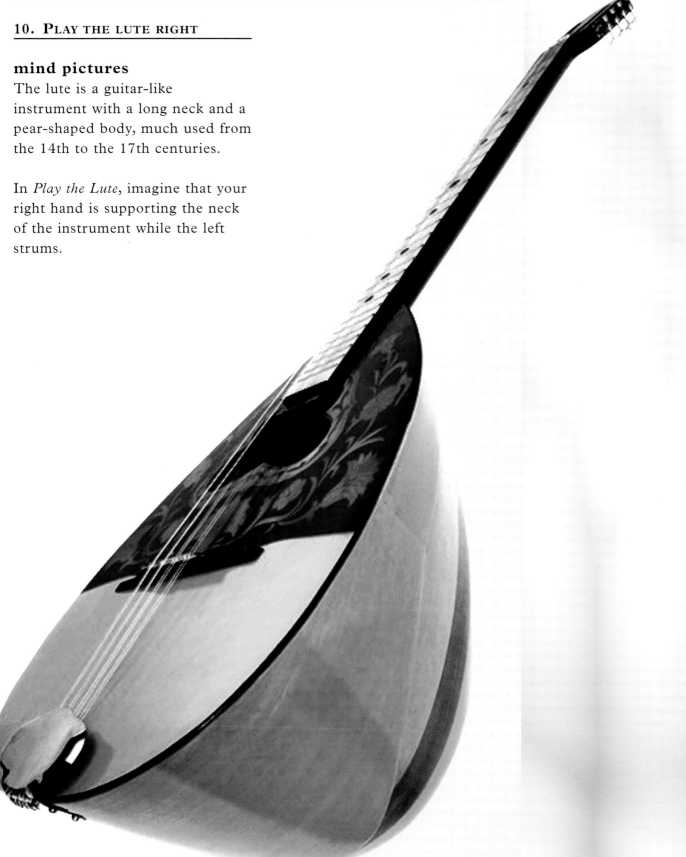

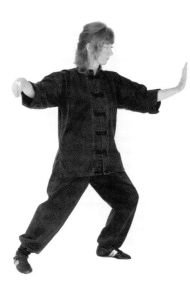

legs and feet

Seventy-five per cent of the weight is taken on the right foot, while raising the ball of the left foot, leaving the heel on the ground.

Bring most of your weight on to your left foot, as you lower it flat to the ground and turn it in towards the right foot. At the same time raise your right heel so that you can straighten your right foot to be in line with your left foot.

Keep most of your weight on your left foot, bending the knee slightly.

body

As your weight goes on to your left foot, turn your body to the right so that you are facing out, over your right foot.

arms and hands

Open your right hand from the hook in which it finished 9. *Single Whip to the Left*.

Keeping it up level with your face, turn your hand and palm to face outward, away from you. Drop your left arm and open it out, forwards and to the left until it is level with your left hip. Keep the palm open, with your fingers

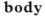

straight and slightly splayed. In one continuous movement, swing it back in towards you body and up in front of your chest, elbow bent, palm facing out.

As you move your weight on to your left foot, and complete the move with your left hand, bring your open right hand down to shoulder level. Turn your palm so that it faces left, fingers still pointing ahead.

Move your left arm across so that the fingers point to your right elbow. As you finish moving it, turn your wrist so that your palm faces down while your fingers continue to point at your right elbow.

Complete the move by sweeping your left hand down to your left hip once again to strum the lute.

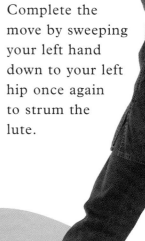

putting it all together

This rather complex move is best achieved by first learning the foot and body movements. Once these have been mastered, you can learn the arm movements separately. When you are happy that you have achieved the correct flowing action, you can put them all together.

essentials

As the lute is played, ensure that all your weight has been moved to your left leg. Keep it there, with the left knee slightly bent and the right leg almost straight. Avoid the temptation to look at the lute you are playing. Keep your head erect, and eyes straight ahead.

breathing

This movement differs from most of the others in that there are two inhalations and two exhalations of breath. This again gives some indication of the pace at which the movements should be made.

Breathe in at the start, as you lower your left hand. The breath should be completed and you should be exhaling as your arm swings back up.

The second intake of breath is taken as you bring your right arm to its final position. Finally breathe out as you lower your left hand at the end of the move.

let your chi flow

Experience the chi flowing through your arms and hands as they move in coordination. The energy will be expressed at different times in the two hands as your arms move. As you try to see and feel yourself in each action, you will feel the chi flowing through each hand in turn.

possible problems

Again the difficulty here is the coordination of the movements, all of which should occur at the same time. Keep in your mind the image of the lute as you are holding it. This will give you the relative positions of your two hands and their distance from your body.

11. STEP WITH SHOULDER STROKE

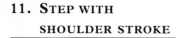

mind pictures

The image here is that you are going to try to push something away, using your right shoulder, rather in the way that you might nudge someone.

legs and feet

This is another situation in which you need to move your feet, hence the mention of the step in its name.

Initially you should take 90 per cent of your weight on your left foot. Draw your right foot closer without lifting it, sweeping the ball of your foot along the ground.

This position is held until the first arm movements are completed.

Then your right foot should be lifted and moved out in a wide stance with most of your weight transferred to it. Bend the right knee slightly more than in the upright position so that you are able to put more of your weight on to it. Remember to keep your left knee slightly bent and the legs relaxed with no tension in them.

body

As you step out widely to the right, keep your body turned slightly to the left. Then twist even more to the left, as you move your left arm, so that you are leading with your right shoulder – making the push.

arms and hands

The right arm is lowered until it hangs straight in front of your body, hand level with your hips, palm turned in, fingers pointing down.

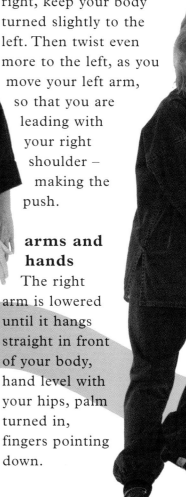

At the same time bend your left arm at the elbow, and sweep your left hand up and across your body, as high as your right shoulder. Then arc it back down close to your right elbow, fingers straight, palm facing down.

Finally, without moving your arm, bend your right wrist so as to bring your right hand up in front of your hip.

putting it all together

All the moves are made at the same time – legs, feet arms and hands – so that it becomes one sweeping action in a very traditional Tai Chi movement. Not only is this beautiful to observe, but you will find it a very satisfying balletic movement to create.

essentials

Although this is described as a shoulder push, your body should remain upright throughout. The push should only come from the twist of the torso.

breathing

Start the arm movements as you breathe in, then breathe out as you complete the arm and leg movements and take your weight on your right foot.

let your chi flow

As you move your hands and arms, you should feel the chi connection between them, as though there was a length of elastic fastened between your hands. Then you should feel the chi surging through your right foot as you complete the move.

possible problems

Initially you may have difficulty in keeping your spine upright while pushing with your shoulder. This will come with practice. Remember to maintain a space between your arms and your body.

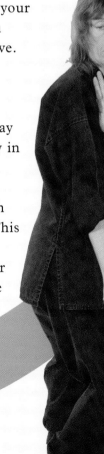

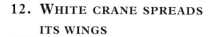

12. WHITE CRANE SPREADS ITS WINGS

mind pictures

As the name suggests, in this position you represent a crane spreading its wings to dry. Your arms will be the wings and you should feel the warm sun drying your feathers as you relax into this stance. Remember that the crane is a large bird, so its heavy wings will move steadily and majestically.

legs and feet

For this movement you start by again moving most of your weight back on to one foot – this time your right. As you do this, allow your left heel to rise so that only the ball and toes are resting on the ground. This foot position is held throughout the following arm movements.

body

As you take up the leg stance, turn your body so that you are facing forwards. Again this position is held throughout the move.

arms and hands

Keep your left hand at your side and bring your right hand up, palm facing out, until it is in front of and slightly above the top of your head.

Now allow your left hand and arm to float out, sideways, level with your left hip, fingers pointing away from you, palm down. Hold both arms outstretched for a few seconds before going on to the next step in this form.

putting it all together

All the movements here are completed simultaneously.

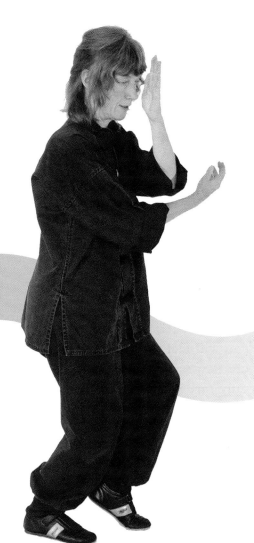

essentials

Lean back while keeping your spine straight and upright. Open out your arms in an unrestrained display, just as the crane would open its wings. At the same time, remember to keep your right knee slightly bent, although it is taking most of your weight.

breathing

Breathe in as you open your arms and out while you are still holding that position. This will indicate to you how long the actual movements take and how long the final position should be held.

let your chi flow

While doing the *White Crane Spreads its Wings* you will feel the chi flowing not only through your hands but also along the whole length of your spine, from your coccyx to your skull.

possible problems

If you do not feel the chi flowing then you are not coordinating the movements correctly. Once you have established the harmonisation of the movements you will know that you have overcome the main problem that this move can present.

There are several reasons why you may not feel the chi flowing. The main one is that, because this appears to be a stretching movement, you lock your arms at the elbows. Keep them very slightly bent.

The second reason is that your right arm is too crooked, blocking the flow of chi. Extend the arm so that your hand is just above your head. Again, you will know when you have found the correct position.

Finally, the chi will not flow as it should if you hold your hands too close to your body. Open up your arms to welcome the sun in a truly expansive gesture.

13. Brush left knee and push

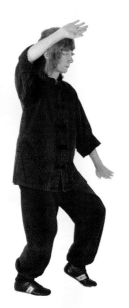

mind pictures

The idea behind this movement is directly linked to the original combative origins of Tai Chi. First, imagine that you are intercepting a blow to your left side, then push your adversary off-balance with your right hand.

legs and feet

With most of your weight on the right foot, slide your left foot out and forward diagonally so that only your left toes and the ball of your foot are touching the ground.

As the second arm movements are made, move three-quarters of your weight forward on to your left foot.

body

Initially the body is turned to the right. Then, as you move your arms, turn it back to the left.

arms and hands

From the previous movement – *12. White Crane Spreads its Wings* – lower your right hand, keeping it close to your body so that it brushes past your breastbone close to your left elbow.

Move your left hand up until it is level with your face, the palm facing right, fingers pointing up.

Continue to sweep down your body with your right hand. At the same time bring your left hand across your chest.

When your right hand reaches your hip level, let it continue the flowing movement out and up, so that it comes back up, level with your face.

Meanwhile your left hand should be allowed to sweep down, brushing your left leg as it does so.

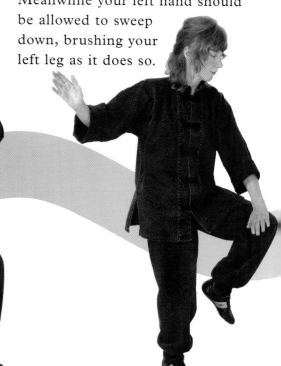

Now turn your right palm out, away from you and straighten your right arm as though pushing someone away, leaning slightly forward as you do so. Be careful not to straighten the arm and thus lock your elbow. Allow it to remain slightly bent and, at the same time, relaxed.

putting it all together

The first body movement is made at the same time as the first arm movements. Then the weight transfer, body and further arm movements are all made simultaneously.

essentials

It is vital to keep your spine and head upright throughout the body movements and during the pushing.

breathing

The inhalation is made as you move your arms into the first position and the breath is allowed out as you lean forward and push.

let your chi flow

You should first feel the chi in your left hand when you bring it up to your face. Next you will feel it in your right hand as this is lowered to your hip. You should then feel it again in your left hand as it brushes your leg and finally again in your right hand as you push.

possible problems

The difficulty with this movement is in the final part where you move the weight, brush and push all at the same time and in one graceful flow. With all the arm movements it is easy to make the mistake of either bending your elbows too tightly and restricting the flow of chi, or straightening your arms and locking the elbows.

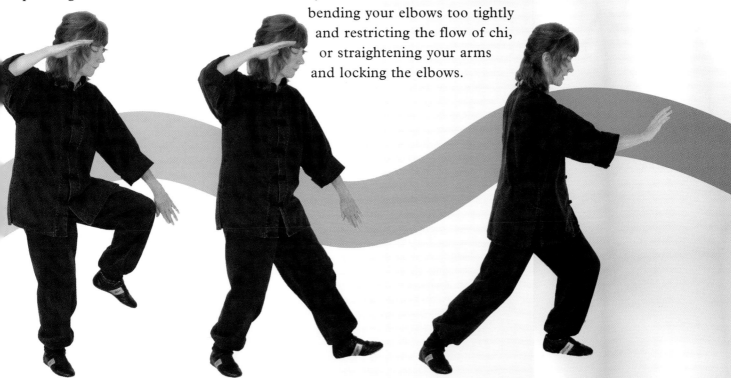

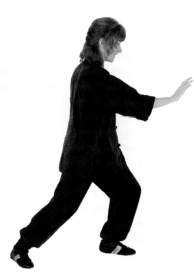

14. PLAY THE LUTE LEFT

mind pictures
The imagery here is exactly as it was in *Play the Lute Right*, except that you are now supporting the neck of the instrument in your left hand while your right hand strums.

legs and feet
Seventy-five per cent of the weight is taken on the left foot, while raising the ball of your right foot, leaving the heel on the ground.

Bring most of your weight on to your right foot, as you lower it flat to the ground and turn it in towards the left foot. At the same time raise your left heel so that you can straighten your left foot to be in line with your right foot.

Keep most of your weight on your right foot, bending the knee slightly.

body
As your weight goes on to your right foot, turn your body to the left so that you are facing out, over your left foot.

arms and hands
Keeping your left hand at chest level turn your palm to face outward, away from you.
Drop your right arm and open it out, forwards and to the right until it is level with your right hip. Keep the palm open, with your fingers straight and slightly splayed.

In one continuous movement swing it back in towards you body and up in front of your chest, elbow bent, palm facing out.

As you move your weight on to your right foot, and complete the move with your right hand, bring your open left hand to shoulder level and turn your palm so that it faces right, fingers still pointing ahead.

Move your right arm across so that the fingers point to your left elbow. As you finish moving it across, turn your wrist so that your palm faces down while your fingers continue to point at your left elbow.

Complete the move by sweeping your right hand down to your left hip once again to strum the lute.

putting it all together

If you have already mastered *Play the Lute Right* you should find no difficulty in putting its mirror image together.

essentials

Remember that all your weight has been moved to your right leg. Keep it there, with the right knee slightly bent and the left leg almost straight. Again, avoid the temptation to look at the lute you are playing. Keep your head erect, and eyes straight ahead.

breathing

This movement is different from most of the others in that there are two inhalations and two exhalations of breath. This again gives some indication of the pace at which the movements should be made.

Breathe in at the start, as you lower your right hand. The breath should be completed and you should be breathing out as your arm swings back up.

The second intake of breath is taken as you bring your left arm to its final position. Finally breathe out as you lower your right hand at the end of the move.

let your chi flow

Experience the chi flowing through your arms and hands as they move in coordination. The energy will be expressed at different times in your two hands as your arms move. As you try to see and feel yourself in each action, you will feel the chi flowing there.

possible problems

As was mentioned previously, the difficulty here is the coordination of the movements, all of which should occur at the same time. Keep in your mind the image of the lute you are holding, as this will give you the relative positions of your two hands and their distance from your body.

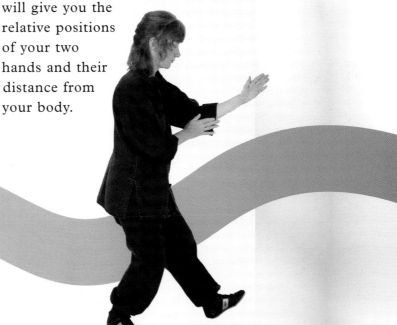

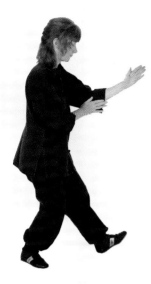

15. BRUSH LEFT KNEE
AND PUNCH

mind pictures

This movement starts exactly as in *13. Brush Left Knee and Push* but then, instead of pushing your opponent away with your right hand, you punch him.

legs and feet

With most of your weight on the right foot, slide your left foot out and forward diagonally so that only your left toes and the ball of your foot are touching the ground.

As the second arm movements are made, move three-quarters of your weight forward on to your left foot.

body

Initially the body is turned to the right. As you move your arms, turn it back and then to the left.

arms and hands

From the previous movement – *14. Play the Lute* – lower your right hand, keeping it close to your body so that it brushes past your breastbone close to your left elbow.

Move your left hand up until it is level with your face, the palm facing right, fingers pointing up.

Continue to sweep down your body with your right hand and at the same time bring your left hand across your chest.

When your right hand reaches your hip level, let it continue the flowing movement out and up, so that it comes back up, level with your face.

Meanwhile your left hand should be allowed to sweep down, brushing your left leg as it does so.

Make a soft fist with your right hand as you turn your palm to face left. Push your fist forward, at heart height. Hold back the punch before your arm is fully extended, leaning forward as you do so.

putting it all together

The first body movement is made at the same time as the first arm movements. Then the weight transfer, body and further arm movements and punch are all made simultaneously.

essentials

Remember that you should keep your spine and head upright throughout the body movements and during the pushing. Be careful not to straighten the arm and lock your elbow when you punch.

breathing

The inhalation is made as you move your arms into the first position and the breath is allowed out as you lean forward and push.

let your chi flow

First you will feel the chi in your left hand when you bring it up to your face. Next you will feel it in your right hand as this is lowered to your hip. You should then feel it again in your left hand as it brushes your leg and finally again in your right hand as you punch.

possible problems

The difficulty with this movement is in the final part where you move the weight, brush and punch all at the same time and in one graceful flow. With all the arm movements it is easy to make the mistake of either bending your elbows too tightly and restricting the flow of chi, or straightening your arms and locking the elbows. Repetition of this move will help you to attain the fluid movement required and enable you to detect the flow of chi more easily.

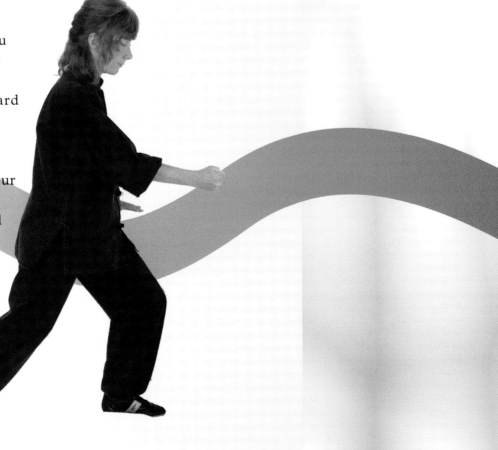

16. Needles at the bottom of the sea

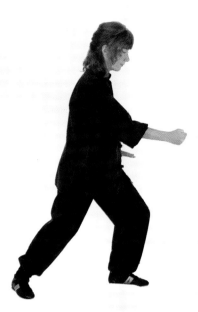

mind pictures

The imagery here is all in the title. You are going to pick up some needles from the ocean floor. The action is imagined to be all under water, which will help to remind you that the movements are made in a steady, flowing, unhurried manner.

legs and feet

Move three-quarters of your weight on to your left foot. Bring your right foot forward, pointing the toe and raising your heel off the ground.

After you have moved your hands, transfer your weight back onto your right foot and raise your left heel. Then bend your knees and sink down keeping all your weight on your right leg.

Straighten your legs and return to an upright posture after you have scooped up the needles.

body

This is one movement where you move your spine from the vertical position. Try not to bend the back so much as tilt your spine forward from the pelvis.

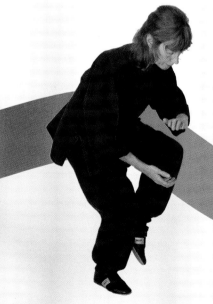

arms and hands

Move your right hand up, out and across your body, with the palm facing to the left. It should finish at about waist height.

Now move your left hand similarly up, out and across your body. It should be slightly higher than your right hand, with the palm resting on your right wrist.

As you bend your knees and sink down, allow your two hands to move down lower, in line with your right leg.

Move your hands even lower by leaning your trunk forward, until your hands are as near to the ground as you can comfortably manage.

Scoop up the imaginary needles from the seabed using your left hand and finish off by slowly returning to the Wu Chi position.

putting it all together

This simple movement is a good one to move a lot of chi if done correctly. After the initial leg movement, all the arm and hand movements should be made simultaneously.

essentials

As you bend forward allow your head to follow the movement instead of looking at the horizon. To do so would put considerable strain on your neck. This is one occasion where you should watch what your hands are doing.

breathing

Finish taking a breath in before you start the movement, then allow your breath out as you bend forward. Resume breathing in as you return to the vertical.

let your chi flow

As mentioned earlier, a lot of chi is generated and moved by this combination of actions. Initially you will feel the chi in your legs and then in both hands as you bring them together.

Feel the final surge of chi as you scoop up the needles from the seabed.

possible problems

The main difficulty here is in keeping your spine straight and yet relaxed as you bend forward. This is the only occasion in the Short Form where you do this, so it is a good idea to practise the movement until you feel the chi flow freely and know that you have got it right.

There are so many benefits from the actions involved in picking up needles from the bottom of the sea that it is well worthwhile to repeat it, using mirror image movements so that you pick up the needles with your right hand. Don't forget to also put all your weight on your right leg.

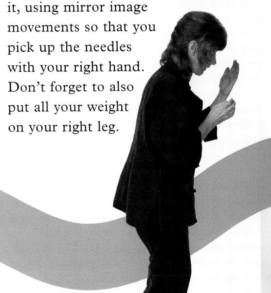
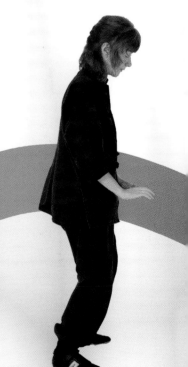

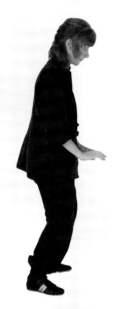

17. WAVE HANDS LIKE CLOUDS

This classic movement is one that we imagine as being typical of Tai Chi when we know nothing about it. Oddly enough, not many practitioners include it in the Short Form. This could be because the full version is rather long, complicated and difficult to learn. The one movement used here is shortened, but still retains the beauty and value of the full version.

mind pictures

You have been levitated above the earth so that you are level with the white fluffy clouds that surround you. You can manipulate these clouds as you wish by taking them in your arms and moving them. As you do so, you describe the shape of the clouds with your hands.

legs and feet

While waving your hands like clouds, you also move your feet along a straight line to your right. Walking, in Tai Chi, has been described as 'walking like a cat'. If you watch a cat as it glides along, stalking its prey, you will know what is meant. Each footfall should be made as though you were stepping on to eggshells that would break if you moved incautiously.

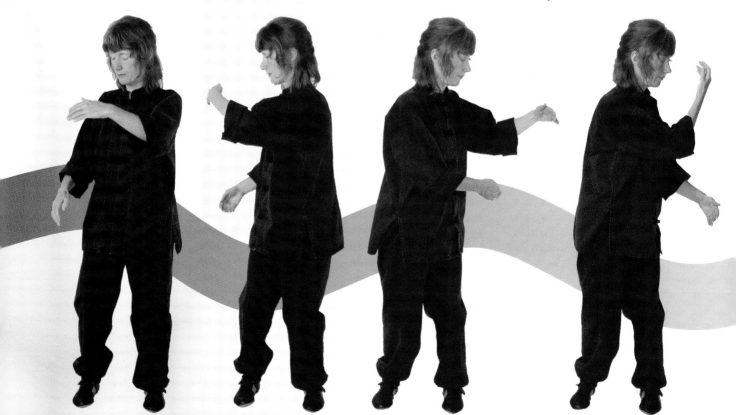

From the previous movement –
*16. Needles at the Bottom of the
Sea* – you have already returned
to the Wu Chi position. Now
taking all your weight on your
left foot, lift your right foot
further away until your feet are
approximately one-and-a-half
shoulder widths apart. Then
distribute your weight equally
between your two feet.

After making the first arm
movements, place all your weight
on your right foot and lift your left
leg, drawing it back to one
shoulder width from your right.

As the second set of arm movements
is being completed, again take your
weight on your left foot and lift your
right foot further away until your feet
are again one-and-a-half shoulder
widths apart. Again you should
redistribute your weight equally
between your two feet. Finally, as the
arm movements are completed, lift
your left foot in again until it is one
shoulder width from your right.

body
Turn your trunk to the left as you
take the weight on your left foot,
and swing it round to the right
when your weight is moved there.
This is repeated with the second
set of leg movements.

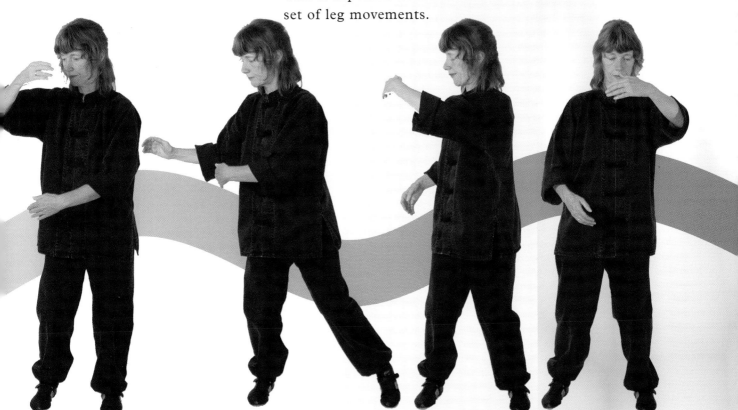

arms and hands

Bring your right hand up and out in front of you, bending your elbow until your hand is level with your face, palm facing down. Move your left arm forward and up towards your body at waist level, turning your wrist so that your palm now faces upwards. You will realise that this leaves your hand and arms in a very similar position to that used in *'holding the ball.'*

As you step and turn to the right, move your right hand out away from your body and down as though moving it round the outer edge of the ball. At the same time move your left hand in towards your body and up. It takes up the mirror image position of the one that your right hand has just been in.

While you are moving the left arm it is impossible to 'hold the ball'. You should allow your hand to face into your body in a natural way, as it moves, finishing with it facing down, *'holding the ball'*.

Now turn your two palms so that they are facing in, the left palm level with the throat, and the right level with your waist. Swing your shoulders to the right and turn your palms to face one another, again 'holding the ball'.

Complete the movement by rotating your hands again, this time continuing the motion so that the right hand comes up against the body while the left hand goes out and over the ball.

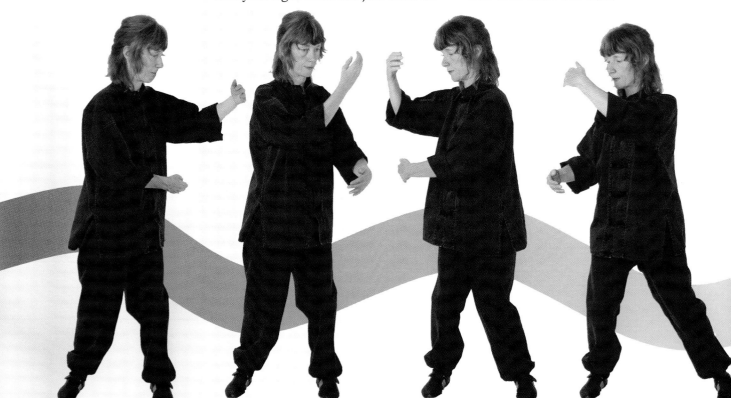

putting it all together

Although this movement sounds complicated, you will see that it can be broken down, rather like ballroom dancing, into the steps and body movements, The steps should coincide with your body swinging left, right, left, right. You will find that the arm movements automatically fit in with these movements.

essentials

Emphasis should be placed on the waist movements that are most important here and are very beneficial to the liver, the digestive and elimination systems. Allow your arms to move easily and freely with the hands floating like the downy clouds that they delineate.

breathing

The breathing gives you the pace at which this movement should be made. Breathe out as you first swing left, then in on turning back right. Repeat the breaths with the repetition of the body movements so that two complete breaths – in and out – are taken from the start to the finish.

let your chi flow

There is a very strong movement of chi while you are doing this exercise. It will be felt in your feet, especially the right foot as you move it and place it down on the ground. Then you will feel it in and between your two hands as they circle one another.

possible problems

Once you have managed to put it all together, the problem is remaining relaxed as you perform the exercise. Be especially careful to keep your waist muscles as loose as possible as there is a tendency for them to tense up as you move your body.

This is another exercise that many instructors will repeat immediately, using the mirror image movements, so that the mid-section of the body is equally exercised on both sides.

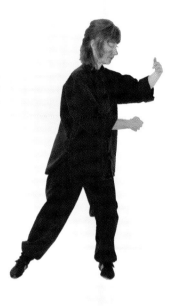

18. FAIR LADY WORKS WITH SHUTTLES

mind pictures

As its name indicates, this is another traditional Tai Chi movement. Imagine that you are weaving with a shuttle held in each hand. Why a 'fair lady' you may ask? First, because weaving with shuttles would be a feminine task and second, it is indicative of the delicacy with which the movements should be made.

The later Western title given to this movement is *'Four Corners'*.

legs and feet

Start by moving 75 per cent of your weight on to your left foot, raising the heel of your right foot as you do so. As your left arm rises, move your weight back so that it is evenly distributed between both feet.

Again take 75 per cent of your weight on to your left foot, raising the heel of your right foot as you lower your right arm.

Come back to an even distribution of weight between the two feet as you finish the movement.

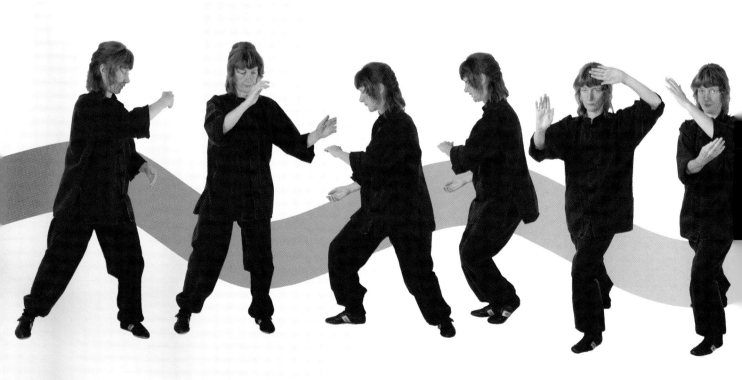

body

The movements of your body follow those of your weight distribution. As you take your weight on your left foot, turn your torso to the left. When your weight is again evenly distributed, swing back to the front. Then repeat the two movements, swinging to the left and then to the front as you lower your right arm and then complete the exercise.

arms and hands

Extend your left hand and arm, straight out, avoiding locking the elbow, until it is shoulder height. At the same time bring your right hand up so that it is level with your waist. Both hands should be pointing forward, palms facing in. Turn your wrist so that your left palm is facing down, and lower your left elbow, drawing your hand closer to your body.

Move your right hand across your body until it is by your left elbow, palm facing up, fingers still extended.

Move your left hand out again and raise it, palm up, until it is at

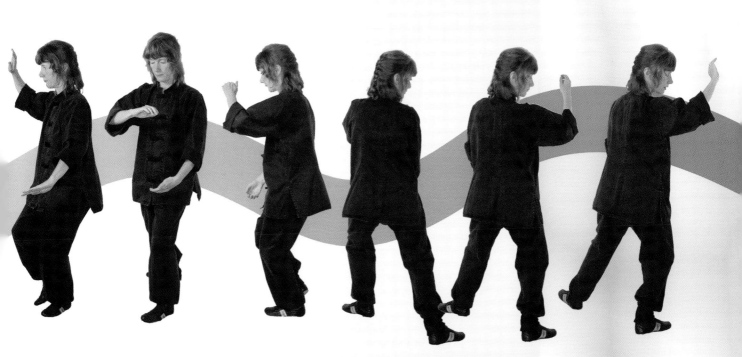

shoulder height, as you move your weight back on to both feet. At the same time move your right arm across so that the fingers point at your left elbow. It is as you complete this movement that you turn to the left again, taking your weight on to your left foot.

Lower your left arm, bent at the elbow, until it is level with your chest, then straighten it out to push your hand forward, being careful not to lock your elbow. At the same time push your right hand up and out so that it is level with your left hand. Keep your palms facing out and fingers pointing up as you bring your weight back on to both feet.

Pull your right arm back, bent so that your right hand again points to your left elbow. As you finish moving your right hand, pull your left elbow down to your waist keeping your hand raised and pointing out.

putting it all together

This is another movement that can be easily broken down into four constituent parts. Try to integrate the feet with the hands and arms as you move your body left, then to the front, left again, and then finish facing forward.

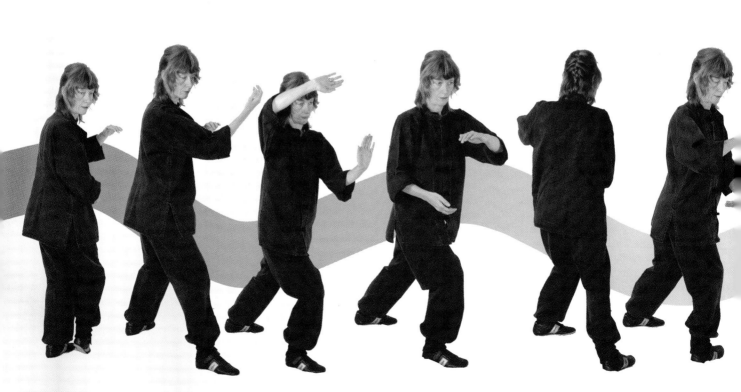

essentials

The hands are important in this exercise as they really dictate what is happening. The lady working with the shuttles would think about where the shuttles were being moved and the rest of her body movements would automatically follow.

breathing

The breathing naturally follows the movements of the feet and body. Start with an intake of breath as you turn to your left and exhale as you come back to the front. Take another breath in as you turn to the left again and exhale as you finish the movement facing the front.

let your chi flow

The chi should be felt strongly flowing up and through the body and out to both arms throughout this movement, especially as the arms are extended.

possible problems

The only difficulty here may be in remembering the movements, which at first may seem rather complex. Do not try to remember all the movements at once. Break the exercise down into simple sections and master each one before moving on to the next.

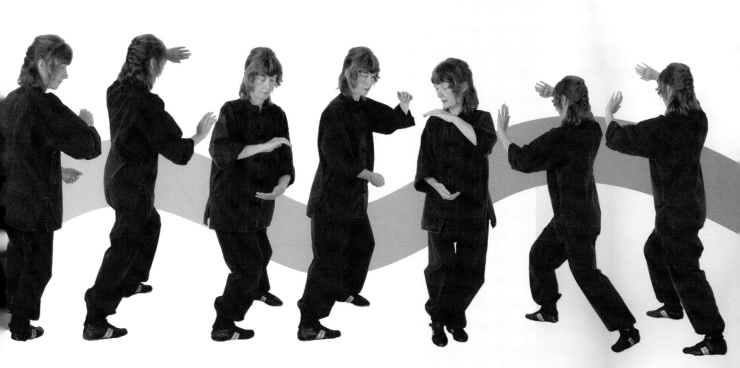

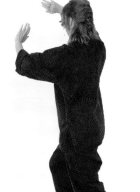

19. FACE THE TIGER AND RETURN TO THE MOUNTAIN

mind pictures

You may consider the connection between the movement and the title even more tenuous in this section. The first part – crossing the hands – is a movement that is traditionally used to repel tigers, during which calm power is demonstrated. The second part is a bodily description of the mountain, high and wide, filling the immediate landscape. This is a nice symmetrical presentation that is easy to learn and perform and yet is a great mover of chi. It represents the first stages of closing down the whole form.

body

Throughout this movement the body and head are kept erect with the eyes looking forward.

arms and hands

Swing both arms forward and up, moving them together so that they cross at the wrists at chin level, palms facing in. The inside of the left wrist should be touching the outside of your right wrist.

Slowly and steadily part your arms, raising them and straightening them as you do so. Keep your palms in, facing you and each other. Remember to leave the arms slightly flexed so as not to lock the elbows.

legs and feet

As you finish the last move – *18. Fair Lady Works with Shuttles* – stand with your weight equally distributed on both feet.

Bend both knees when you have brought your arms down level with them. Slowly bend them more and more until they are as fully bent as is comfortable. Then straighten back up again as your arms are finally raised.

Continue the movement of both arms, in a large arc out and down until they are level with your knees.

As you bend your knees, let your arms descend so that you end up in a sitting pose with your hands shoulder-width apart, just above your knees.

Turn your palms upwards and, as you stand upright again, raise your hands, palms up, until they are level with your waist.

putting it all together

All is simple until that last movement where you straighten up and raise your hands. At this point you should imagine that you are lifting a great weight. Feel the load trying to press your arms down as you lift them up.

essentials

Lowering your body steadily, while bending your knees, try to remain upright and yet relaxed and looking straight ahead.

breathing

Take an in-breath before you start and let it go out as you sink down. Breathe in again as you come back up to the Wu Chi position.

let your chi flow

A great deal of chi is generated with this simple movement. Feel it being expressed through your arms as they circle, through your legs and feet as you go down, and strongly through your arms, as you have to exert the energy to lift them up.

possible problems

There are two possible sources of difficulty here. You may find it difficult to keep your shoulders relaxed as your arms circle and also at the end of the movement where you push up with your hands. Similarly it may sound impossible to keep your legs relaxed while bending your knees. The secret is to let it happen. Feel the movements as they occur and let your arms and legs float.

20. CLOSE

mind pictures

This short movement brings you to the end of your Form and you are, literally, closing down. You are coming back home, grounding yourself, in mind, body and spirit, ready to return to the material world.

legs and feet

Initially your legs and feet are in the Wu Chi position with your weight equally distributed between them. At the end of the movement, both feet are drawn together, sliding your left foot in against your right.

body

Throughout this move your body should remain still and erect.

arms and hands

Raise both arms in front of you, keeping them at shoulder width and extending them, palms down, until you are reaching ahead, without locking your elbows. You should finish with your hands at shoulder height.

Keeping your palms facing the ground, slowly push down as though you are deflating a large balloon. Continue pushing down until your arms are just in front of you, as low as they will go.

Let your wrists relax and bring your hands back to your sides in the Wu Chi position.

putting it all together

There should be no problem with coordinating the movements here.

essentials

If anything, take these movements more slowly than usual. Imagine that as you come to the end of this Short Form you are winding down.

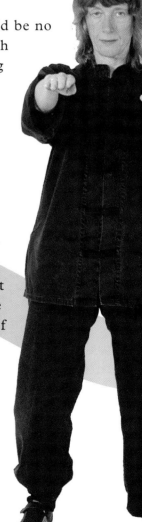

When you have completed the movements, stand still for a few moments, giving your internal energies time to balance and flow before moving off.

breathing

Breathe in as you raise your arms and out as you let them sink back down. Then take several calming breaths as you remain motionless after the final movement.

let your chi flow

The chi flows strongly through your hands and arms during this closing movement, until the last movement with your feet. Then you will feel it flow through your legs and feet, into the earth to ground you.

possible problems

Don't be tempted to rush these movements because they are so simple and easy to execute. Allow the chi to flow for as long as possible. Don't move off until you are completely grounded.

This completes the Short Form. It will have taken you much less time to complete than it does to read.

You have completed 20 movements that have exercised equally almost all the upper parts of your body. In order to simplify things for the beginner, you will find that I have used those movements that require the least foot and leg action. These will come later when you progress to a Long Form.

All of the above movements can be duplicated using their mirror images and quite often forms are shown that include these repetitions.

This Short Form is one of many that range from as few as a dozen moves to well over 30. The Long Forms, usually starting with the Short Form, extend to make a total of some 50 moves.

You will find that all teachers have their own Forms. It is simply a matter of personal preference as to which moves are included, which are left out and in what order they are combined.

WORKING WITH A PARTNER

If you worked with a partner to learn the basic positions, you can now work together in some simple shared exercises. As you will see, this is not the type of workout that you can do on your own. One benefit you will both gain is that your movements become smoother and more subtle as each of you is able to anticipate the intention of the other. These simple actions will also help you to become and remain more alert and well balanced.

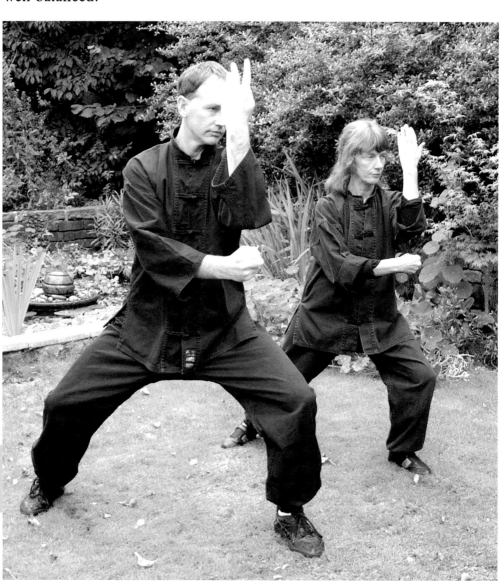

Right: the Long Yang second set.

If you wish, you can consider these as warming-up exercises to get you into a harmonious frame of mind with your partner before executing the Form.

POLISH THE WINDOWS

1. Stand comfortably relaxed with your left foot advanced about 12 inches (30 cm) in front of the right, and shoulder-width apart.

2. Have your partner stand similarly, facing you, so that your two left feet are level at the toes.

3. You should both raise both hands, palms facing out, and place them together, palm to palm, shoulder-width apart.

4. Without moving your torso, start to move your co-joined hands in a circular motion. The movement should not be strained or forced, but the hands should move out to the side so that your left hand is where your right started, and vice-versa as you circle.

5. Keep the circle flowing for about 15 seconds, then revolve your hands in the opposite direction. Both partners should maintain a firm and constant pressure with both hands.

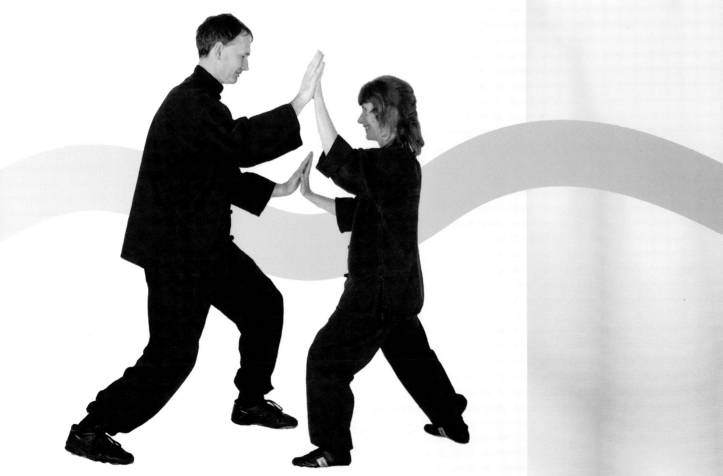

SAW WOOD

1. Stand facing one another as in the previous exercise – left foot advanced.

2. Place your right palms together, directly in front of and between you, keeping your left hands by your sides.

3. Increase the pressure between your two hands and push your partner's arm back. Your partner should allow this to happen, though still maintaining pressure, until their upper arm is pushed back level with their side. Breathe out steadily as your arm moves forward.

4. As you move forward, raise your right heel and transfer your weight on to your left foot.

5. Your partner should move their weight back to their right foot, raising the ball of their left foot as they do so. At this point they should be breathing in.

6. Decrease the pressure on your partner's palm as they increase the pressure on yours.

7. Move back to your original position, breathing in as you do so, until you are back on your right foot and your partner's weight is forward on to their left foot. They breathe out as they make the forward movement.

8. Their arm and hand continue to push your arm back until your arm is level with your side, and then the whole cycle is repeated.

9. This exercise should be repeated for about 15 seconds. Then change your stance to right feet forward, change to left hands doing the sawing and repeat the cycle.

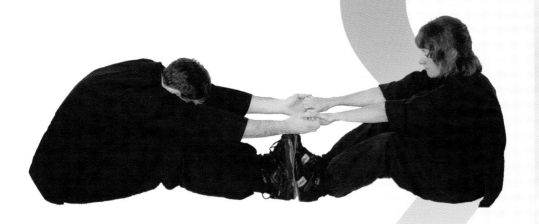

SEE-SAW

This is an exercise that you will see children doing just for the fun of it.

1. You and your partner should sit down on the floor, facing one another so that the soles of your feet are touching and you both have your legs slightly bent, shoulder-width apart, knees raised.

2. Grasp each other's hands by hooking your fingers together.

3. Start the see-saw by one of you leaning back, pulling as you do so, while the other allows him/herself to lean forward.

4. As you lean back, breathe in and as you lean forward, breathe out.

5. Maintain a steady backwards and forwards motion, being careful not to strain your back.

6. At the same time, try to maintain some resistance against being pulled forward, but avoid the tendency to straighten your legs.

7. Again, continue steadily for 15 seconds before taking a rest.

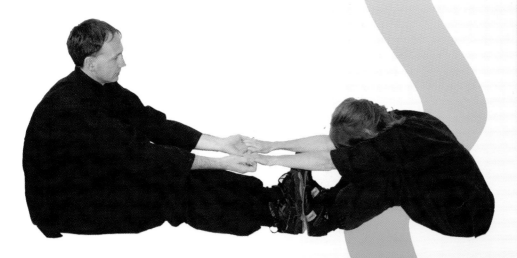

STICKY HANDS

Here is an exercise that is not strictly Tai Chi but is a useful way to increase your sensitivity and awareness of movement.

1. Stand facing your partner who should stretch their right hand towards you, palm facing down.

2. Place your right hand, palm flat down, on top of your partner's and close your eyes.

3. Your partner should now slowly move their hand left and right. This should not be a rhythmic movement, but should change direction suddenly though smoothly.

4. At this stage you will be able to follow their movements easily. Do so and try to anticipate when they will change direction.

5. Now have your partner move their hand steadily up and down. Again try to follow their movements. At first you will have difficulty in anticipating when they move their hand down and away from yours, but with practice you will find that you can do this.

6. Next have your partner combine the up and down movements with the side to side in any random pattern.

7. When you are used to these movements, have your partner move steadily around the room. This includes moving you sideways, backwards, forwards and diagonally. Have them move steadily, with smooth gliding movements appropriate to Tai Chi.

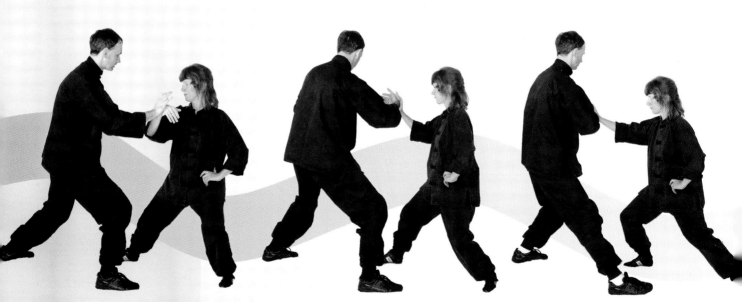

8. Follow them and again try to anticipate when they will change direction and which direction they will take.

9. When you have exhausted the possibilities, change over and let your partner try the same exercise.

This exercise is very simple – children are extremely good at it. You will find that you need to concentrate on two levels: First, on the actual hand movements and second, on trying to anticipate your partner's next move. The best results are obtained if you can remain relaxed mentally and physically the whole time that your eyes are closed.

If you find this exercise difficult initially, try doing it to music. Choose rather slow, rhythmical music and you will find that this helps.

After some practice, you will find that eventually you become more sensitive to the course of the energy currents in your partner, as though you are in tune with one another. As a result the two of you will move round the floor like a couple dancing.

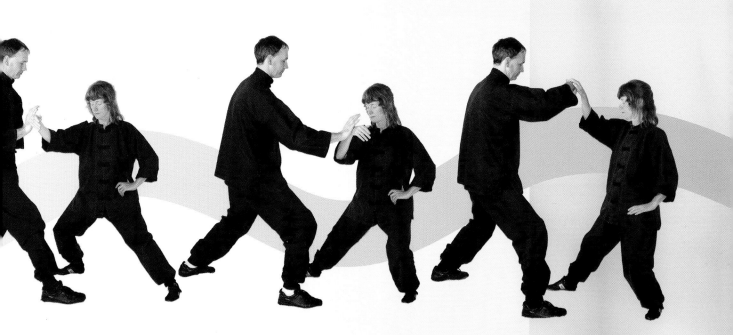

AND FINALLY...

Y ou have now come to the end of this book. I hope that it has inspired you to start out on a new venture. This project could alter your life, for ever. The main difficulty with taking up a new way of life is that you have to rethink it. Instead of struggling along with no life-plan, you have to start over and apply yourself in an ordered way.

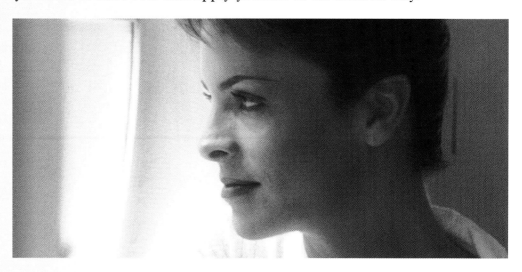

First you have to make the decision to practise Tai Chi regularly. Then you need to appreciate that the changes you are looking for will take time to appear. There will be no obvious change in your mind, body or spirit after one session of Tai Chi. Change will come slowly, and at first you may not even realise it is happening. It is only when you are able to look back after many sessions that you will see and appreciate the transformation that has come about.

If you take up Tai Chi then you will realise that it affects your whole being – for the good. You will find that your Tai Chi – and it will be your own – is very personal and private. It is about you, your body, your mind and your spirit. You will realise that you don't just 'do' Tai Chi – you enter in to it. You become part of it, just as much as it becomes part of you.

As the Chinese would say – you enter into The Way. The important thing about The Way is that it is all. The journey is the destination. You are not seeking an end goal, just the way.

Eventually you will discover, through Tai Chi, what is essential to your life and what can be discarded. You will find yourself.

May good fortune attend you all your days.

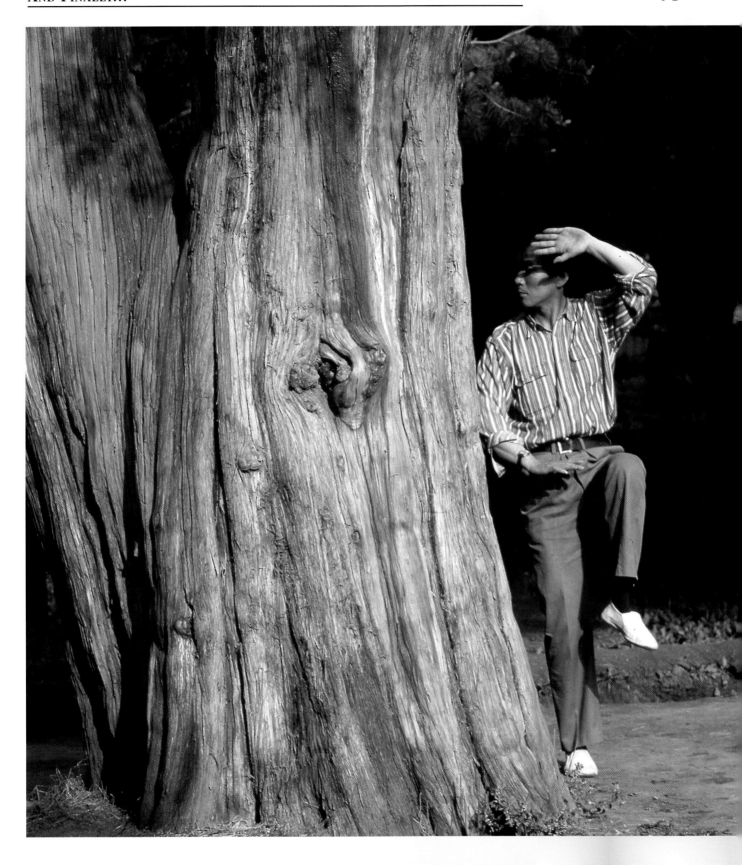

FURTHER READING

Brecher, Paul, Master Earl Montague – Principles of Tai Chi – HarperCollins.

Chuckrow, Robert – The Tai Chi – Paul H Crompton.

Chuen, Master Lam Kam – Step-by-step Tai Chi – Gaia Books.

Clark, Angus – Tai Chi: the Complete Illustrated Guide – Element Books.

Crompton, Paul – Tai Chi for Two: The Practice of Push Hands – Paul Crompton Ltd.

The Healing Art of Tai Chi – Sterling.

Liebermann, Loni – The Foldout Book of Tai Chi Chuan – Weatherhill Publishers.

Little, John R. (editor) & Wong, Curtis (editor) – Ultimate Guide to Tai Chi – Contemporary Books Inc.

Man-ch'ing C. & Smith R. – Tai-chi – Tuttle Publishing.

Parry, Robert – Teach Yourself Tai Chi – Teach Yourself series, Hodder & Stoughton.

Parry, Robert – The Tai Chi Manual – Piatkus Books.

Pawlett, Ray – Beginner's Guide To Tai Chi – D&S Books.

Sutton, Nigel – Applied Tai Chi Chuan – A & C Black.

Tucker, Paul – Tai Chi – Southwater.

Robinson, Ronnie – Tai Chi – Collins Gem Series, Collins.

The Tai Chi Union of Great
Britain
1 Littlemill Drive
Balmoral Gardens
Crookston
Glasgow G53 7GE
Tel 0141 638 2946
Fax 0141 621 1220
E-mail secretary@taichiunion.com

The British Council for Chinese
Martial Arts
C/o 31 Neale Drive
Greasby
Wirral
Merseyside
Liverpool L49 1SE
Tel/Fax 0151 677 4471

Tai Chi Kung Forum for Health
and Special Needs
163 Palatine Road
Didsbury
Manchester M20 2GH

The British Open Tai Chi Ch'uan
Championships
9 Ashfield Road
London N14 7LA
Tel 020 8368 6815

British Tai Chi Chuan & Shaolin
Kung Fu Association
28 Linden Farm Drive
Countesthorpe
Leicester LE8 3SX

Tai Chi Caledonia
18 Branziert Road North
Kilearn
Glasgow G63 9RF
Tel 0131 552 35722

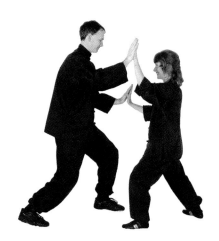